Quit
Ultra-processed Foods
in 4 Weeks

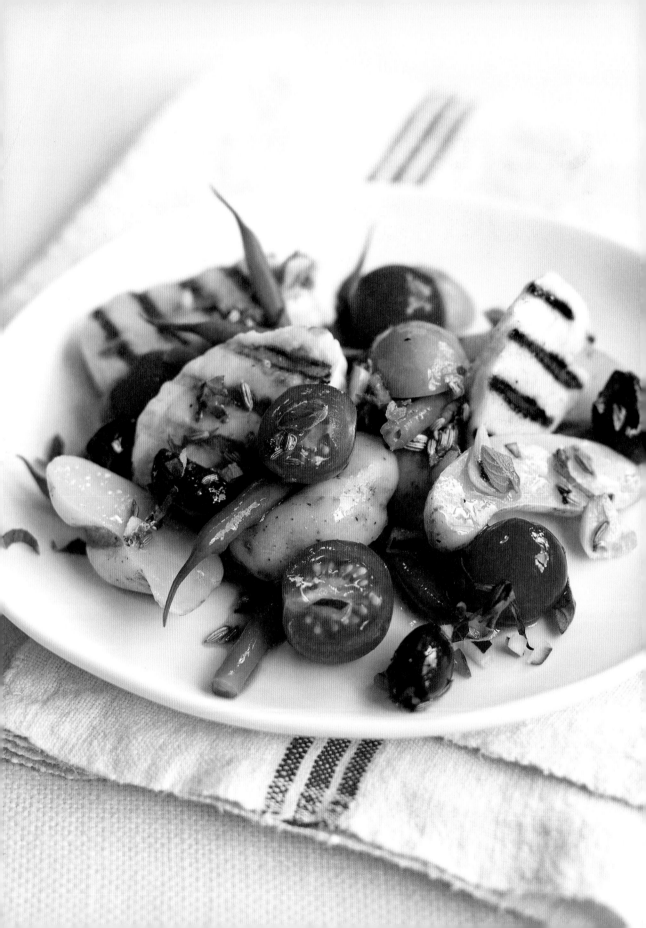

ANGELA DOWDEN

Quit Ultra-processed Foods in 4 Weeks

Simple recipes & meal plans to eat fresh for life

hamlyn

First published in Great Britain in 2024 by Hamlyn,
an imprint of Octopus Publishing Group Ltd
Carmelite House
50 Victoria Embankment
London EC4Y 0DZ
www.octopusbooks.co.uk

An Hachette UK Company
www.hachette.co.uk

Distributed in the US by
Hachette Book Group
1290 Avenue of the Americas
4th and 5th Floors
New York, NY 10104

Distributed in Canada by
Canadian Manda Group
664 Annette St, Toronto,
Ontario, Canada M6S 2C8

ISBN 978-0-600-63851-3

A CIP catalogue record for this book is available from the British Library.

Printed and bound in Italy

10 9 8 7 6 5 4 3 2 1

Editorial Director: Natalie Bradley
Art Director: Yasia Williams
Designer: Geoff Fennell
Senior Editor: Leanne Bryan
Production Manager: Caroline Alberti

Picture credits

Octopus Publishing Group: 111; Stephen Conroy 140, 166, 174; Vanessa Davies 177;
Will Heap 2, 6, 43, 79, 90, 101, 109, 115, 116, 128, 131, 132, 135, 139, 143, 143, 144, 147, 170;
Lis Parsons 16, 40, 51, 63, 64, 67, 72, 75, 84, 89, 93, 96, 99, 105, 106, 119, 120, 123, 124,
154, 158, 173, 181, 182, 186; William Reavell 9, 19, 19, 35, 44, 48, 68, 102, 162, 165, 178;
Craig Robertson 13, 20, 56, 59, 71, 95; William Shaw 31, 32, 36, 39, 47, 52, 60, 76, 80,
83, 112, 136, 153, 161, 185; Ian Wallace 150, 157.

Cookery notes

Standard level spoon measurements are used in all recipes.
1 tablespoon = one 15 ml spoon
1 teaspoon = one 5 ml spoon

Both imperial and metric measurements have been given in all recipes.
Use one set of measurements only and not a mixture of both.

Ovens should be preheated to the specific temperature – if using a
fan-assisted oven, follow manufacturer's instructions for adjusting
the time and the temperature.

Eggs should be medium unless otherwise stated.

This book includes dishes made with nuts and nut derivatives.

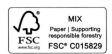

Contents

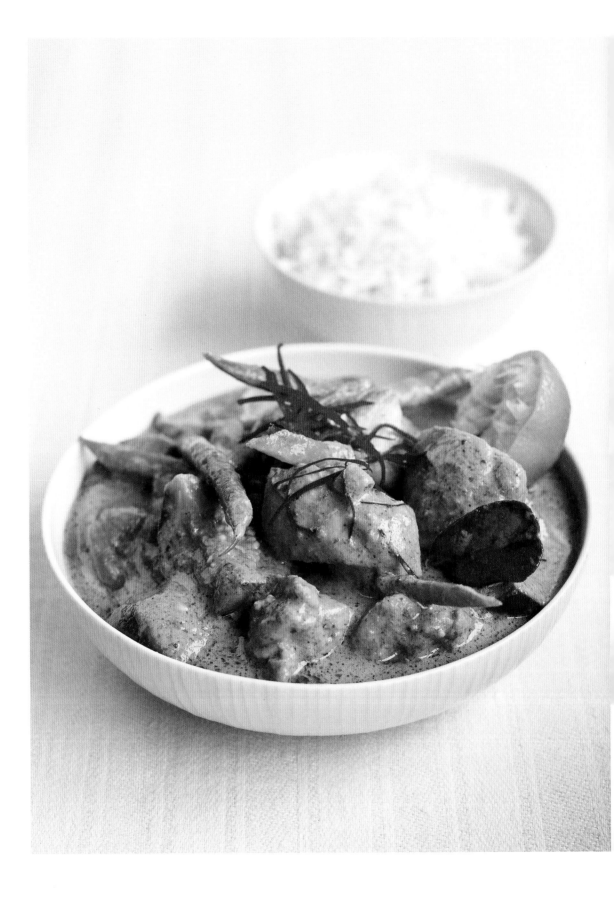

Introduction

You may only have heard of ultra-processed foods or UPFs recently, but this terminology is fast becoming part of our permanent food and nutrition vocabulary. UPFs are convenient, appealing, contain ingredients we won't readily find in our home kitchens, and are often heavily marketed to grab our attention.

Although UPFs may tempt our taste buds, research suggests that they come at a significant cost to our health. UPFs are associated with a higher risk of cardiovascular disease (including heart attacks and strokes), high blood pressure, type 2 diabetes and cancer. People with diets high in UPFs are also likely to consume excess calories and gain weight. Shockingly, ultra-processed foods make up over 50 per cent of the calories we consume in the UK.[1]

However, a 2021 YouGov survey on behalf of the British Nutrition Foundation (BNF) found that many of us struggle to identify UPFs in the foods that we buy.[2] *Quit Ultra-processed Foods in 4 Weeks* will show you how to recognize a UPF and how to make your diet much less reliant on these items. The recipes that follow offer easy and tasty alternatives to UPFs, and the four-week meal planner simplifies the process of choosing less processed food both at home and when on the go.

In just four weeks you will be regularly eating tasty, better quality and more nutritious food, and will have begun reaping the health benefits too.

From unprocessed to ultra-processed: the NOVA classification system

Some level of processing is crucial to the production of a safe, secure and palatable food supply chain. The NOVA classification system groups processed foods into four tiers according to the extent and purpose of the industrial processing they undergo.

Derived from the Portuguese *nova classificação* ('new classification'), NOVA was developed by researchers at the Center for Epidemiological Studies in Health and Nutrition at the University of São Paulo in Brazil in 2009. Though not perfect, NOVA is the most commonly used classification system that researchers and policymakers turn to in order to understand the potential health effects of various foods based on their ingredients.

The four NOVA groups are: [3]

1. Unprocessed and minimally processed foods
2. Processed culinary ingredients
3 Processed foods
4. Ultra-processed foods

1. Unprocessed and minimally processed foods

According to the NOVA system, unprocessed (or natural) foods are things you would immediately recognize as 'whole' foods, such as fruit, vegetables, eggs and simple cuts of meat and fish.

Minimally processed foods are those that have been through 'light-touch' processes such as drying, pasteurizing, grinding, roasting, non-alcoholic fermentation or freezing. Examples include milk and plain yogurt, unsalted nuts, flour, rice and pasta, pulses, dried herbs and spices, dried fruit, pure fruit juice, tea and coffee. These foods do not contain added sugar, fat, oil or salt.

2. Processed culinary ingredients

This group comprises single ingredient foods obtained by slightly more complex industrial processes, such as pressing, centrifuging, refining, extracting or mining. Examples include vegetable, nut and olive oils, vinegar, salt, butter, lard, sugar and molasses from cane or beet, honey and maple syrup, and starches extracted from corn or other plants. NOVA group 2 nutrients are typically used to prepare, season and cook group 1 foods.

3. Processed foods

In most cases, the foods in NOVA group 3 are created when group 2 ingredients (e.g. salt, fats, oil, sugar, etc.) are added to group 1 foods during the manufacturing process in the food industry. This category includes canned foods (fruit, vegetables and fish, including those in syrup or brine), along with traditionally made bread and cheese, tofu, tomato purée, salted nuts, wine and beer. Dry cured ham, bacon and other salted, cured or smoked meat and fish also fall into this group.

These foods are processed, but minimally, and are of less concern than UPFs. Any additives they contain are critical to the process of making the food (e.g. calcium sulphate, which is used as a coagulant in the manufacture of tofu, and curing salts, which are used to make bacon).

4. Ultra-processed foods

These heavily altered foods are the ones we are most interested in and the focus of this book. NOVA group 4 ultra-processed foods are often:

- Ready-to-eat, ready-to-drink or ready-to-heat formulations
- Not recognizable as 'whole' foods
- Calorie dense and high in fats, sugar and salt
- Laced with flavours, colours, sweeteners, preservative emulsifiers and other additives that help make food hyper-palatable (moreish)
- Made with processes that include 'extrusion' (for example, puffed savoury snacks), 'forming' (for example, chicken nuggets) and the chemical modification of fat to alter its melting point and 'mouth feel'.

Commonly consumed ultra-processed foods with low nutritional quality include carbonated drinks, pre-prepared hot dogs and burgers, biscuits, sweets, chocolate bars, ice cream, energy drinks, dehydrated 'instant' meals, sweetened yogurts and savoury snacks.

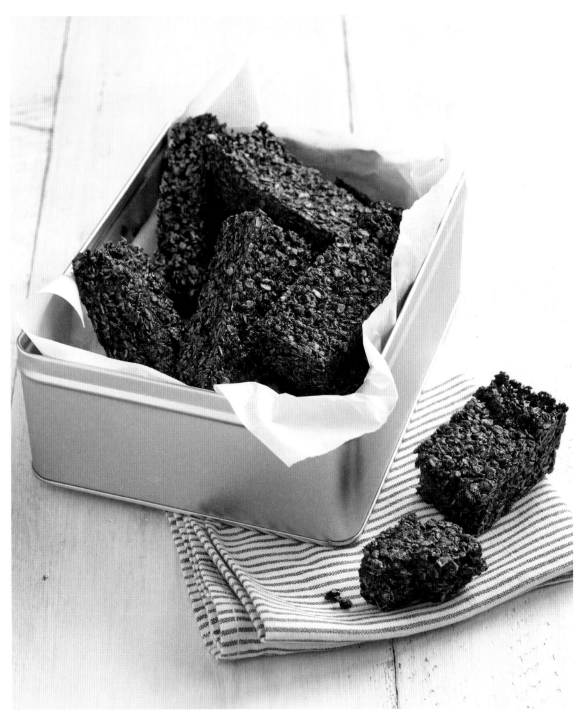

The table below provides a more detailed list of UPFs, along with some examples of less processed alternatives.

UPF category	Examples	Less processed alternatives
Savoury snacks	Flavoured crisps and popcorn; maize/wheat/tortilla/lentil snacks; popped and puffed snacks and crackers	Homemade popped corn; bought popcorn/crisps made with only corn/potatoes, vegetable oil and salt
Soft drinks	Fizzy drinks and fruit squashes (both full sugar and diet/low sugar versions)	Water, fruit juice (or watered-down fruit juice)
Bakery and biscuits	Cakes, brownies, doughnuts, pastries, cookies, biscuits	Homebaked goods such as the Banana and Pecan Loaf on page 160 and the Peach and Brown Sugar Muffins on page 164
Confectionery	Chocolate bars, jelly sweets, boiled sweets, marshmallows, fudge, toffees	Chocolate made with only cocoa mass, sugar, cocoa butter and vanilla
Bars	Cereal bars, protein bars, breakfast bars, energy bars	Homemade granola or flapjacks, such as the Chocolate Flapjacks on page 163
Desserts	Ice cream and other frozen desserts, trifles, jelly, mousses	Fresh or canned fruit and cream
Takeaways and ready meals	Pizzas, curries, lasagne, Chinese and Thai dishes, fast-food burgers; bought sandwiches or wraps; microwave-ready or oven-ready meals	Homemade chicken and vegetable stir-fry; or try the Lasagne on page 125 or the Fiorentina Pizzas on page 88
Breakfast cereals	Most boxed ready-to-eat varieties; some mueslis and granolas	Shredded wheat, porridge made with oats and milk; or try the Maple-glazed Granola with Fruit on page 33

UPF category	Examples	Less processed alternatives
Dairy products and alternatives	Flavoured yogurts, milkshakes, cheese spreads, cheese strings; plant milk alternatives including soya, rice, oat, almond	Plain natural yogurt and lower fat or full-fat milk, non-processed hard cheese and full-fat soft cheese
Processed meat products	Hot dogs, sausages, chicken nuggets, paté, luncheon meat, meat pies	Lean cuts of meat (steak, chicken breast, lamb chop)
Breads, rolls and wraps	Most pre-packaged types found in supermarkets	Any bread made with only flour, water, yeast and salt. Many sourdough loaves are also lower in additives. Or see the Baking chapter on page 149 for homemade ideas
Meat alternatives	Plant-based burgers and sausages (soy, wheat, pea protein, microprotein)	Tofu, plain hummus; or try the Baked Beans on page 49
Potato and vegetable products	Hash browns, waffles, potato croquettes, most oven chips; onion rings, bhajis	Home-cooked baked or mashed potatoes; oven chips made with only potatoes and oil (see the note about vegetable oil on page 18)
Sauces and dressings	Pasta sauces, recipe sauces, stir-fry sauces; salad dressings, mayonnaise; chutneys, pickles; table sauces such as BBQ sauce and tomato ketchup	Passata (made with only tomatoes and salt); homemade vinaigrette – see the Basil Vinaigrette on page 70; or try the Classic Bolognese sauce on page 121
Fish products	Fish fingers, battered/breaded fish; crab sticks	Home-cooked grilled or panko-coated fish; or try the Easy Fish Pie with Crunchy Potato Topping on page 103
Others	Stock cubes, gravy granules, packet recipe mixes; most syrups and sweeteners	Salt, pepper, herbs, homemade stock, sugar, maple syrup, honey

The health impact of ultra-processed foods

Scientific evidence indicates that a high consumption of UPFs can adversely affect a person's health. A major reason is likely to be that these foods tend to be lower in vitamins and fibre, and higher in calories, saturated fat, salt and sugar, which are implicated in conditions such as obesity, heart disease, diabetes and high blood pressure.

There are other factors, however, beyond poor nutritional value, that are thought to make UPFs unhealthy. One of these is that the natural structure (or 'matrix') of the food is often significantly changed through ultra-processing, which may affect the way nutrients are released. For example, flour that is ground very finely will release sugar into your bloodstream faster than flour that still contains pieces of the whole grain.

Ultra-processing often results in softer-textured food too, which can be consumed quickly, meaning you can take on board more calories in a shorter amount of time. Additionally, the 'cosmetic' additives in UPFs – such as flavours, colours, emulsifiers and sweeteners – may have adverse health effects not captured by official safety assessments. These could include inflammation and detrimental effects to the health of your gut microbiota (the microbes that live in your gut that help support your digestion and immune defense).

Most of the research looking into UPFs and disease is associative, so can not prove cause and effect. Nevertheless, there are some compelling studies. Let's take a look at the specific diseases and conditions that consumption of UPFs is linked with.

Cardiovascular disease

In a study published in *The British Medical Journal* (BMJ) in 2019, researchers collected data on the foods consumed by almost 105,000 French people over several 24-hour periods[4]. They then examined the cardiovascular health of these people over a maximum of 10 years.

The results showed that a 10 per cent increase in the proportion of UPFs consumed was associated with a 13 per cent higher rate of coronary heart disease. It was also associated with a 11 per cent higher rate of cerebrovascular disease (strokes, aneurysms, etc.).

In another study, a Chinese meta-analysis of 10 studies involving more than 325,000 men and women, those who ate the most UPFs were 24 per cent more likely to experience cardiovascular problems (heart attacks, strokes and angina) than those who ate the least[5]. The same study found people had the lowest risk of any cardiovascular events when ultra-processed foods made up less than 15 per cent of their calorie intake.

High blood pressure

In a study that tracked 10,000 middle-aged Australian women for 15 years, those with the highest proportion of ultra-processed foods in their diet were 39 per cent more likely to develop high blood pressure than those with the lowest[6].

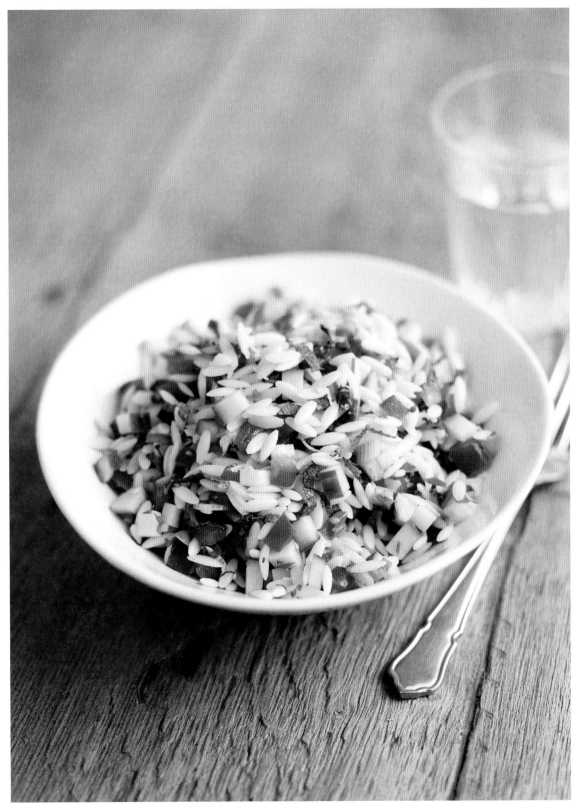

Cancer

A study from Imperial College London found that a higher consumption of UPFs was associated with a greater risk of developing cancer[7]. The researchers collected information on the diets of 200,000 middle-aged adults and monitored their health over a 10-year period. For every 10 per cent increase in ultra-processed foods in a participant's diet, there was a 2 per cent increased incidence in cancers overall. For ovarian cancer specifically, there was a 19 per cent increase, while brain cancer was also disproportionately higher in those with the greatest UPF consumption.

Type 2 diabetes

In a study of 21,800 men and 82,907 women (the same French population as in the cardiovascular health study mentioned on page 12), scientists found that type 2 diabetes rates were nearly one-and-a-half times higher in participants with the highest UPF intake compared with those with the lowest UPF consumptions.[8]

The research suggested that a 10 per cent increase in ultra-processed foods in the diet was linked to a 15 per cent higher risk of type 2 diabetes.

Depression

American researchers who examined data on the diet and mental health of over 30,000 female nurses, found that UPFs were associated with a higher risk of depression or being prescribed antidepressants[9]. The nurses who ate the most ultra-processed foods – nine or more servings per day – had a 50 per cent higher risk of developing depression than those in the bottom fifth of consumers – eating four or fewer servings per day.

Ultra-processed foods and your weight

One small but well-designed study by researchers at the National Institute for Diabetes and Digestive and Kidney Diseases (NIDDK) in Maryland, USA, showed that UPFs can contribute significantly to obesity[10]. The researchers split volunteers into two groups, giving one group an ultra-processed diet and the other group a diet that was only minimally processed. After two weeks the groups switched regimens for another fortnight.

Importantly, the diets were rated as equally enjoyable and matched as closely as possible in terms of calorie, sugar, fat, fibre and micronutrient (vitamin and mineral) content. The subjects were allowed to eat as much as they wanted to feel full.

The results showed that when people were on the UPF diet they ate more calories and gained an average of 2 lb (0.9 kg). Conversely, when they were eating minimally processed food, they ate fewer calories and lost 2 lb (0.9 kg).

This result suggests that something about ultra-processed food – maybe changes to the food matrix or texture as previously discussed – makes it less satiating, so we are more prone to over-eating it.

How to spot a UPF

It's a good idea to get familiar with the UPF examples and their healthier substitutions on page 10. For products you see in the supermarket that you are unsure about, however, here are three telltale signs to watch out for:

1 **Many ingredients** As a very rough guide, if there are more than five ingredients you should dig further as you are probably looking at a UPF or at least at a processed food.

2 **Ingredients you don't recognize as 'food'** If you see sweeteners, preservatives, emulsifiers, thickeners, stabilizers or colours in the ingredients list, this is confirmation you're looking at a UPF. Words such as 'hydrolyzed', 'isolate', 'modified', 'gum', 'formed' and 'shaped' are also unmistakable signals that this is a UPF.

3 **Red traffic lights (or no traffic lights)** Under the nutritional traffic light system, many UPFs will score red for sugar, saturated fat and salt. And no traffic light labelling at all is a potential indicator that a product is a UPF (as traffic lights are voluntary). It probably means the manufacturer isn't keen to shout about the nutritional value of their product.

Ten simple ways to cut down on UPFs

Here are some immediate changes you can make to your shopping and cooking habits to get you started on the right track.

1 Make home-cooked meals as often as you can (look at our four-week meal plans for inspiration and help on establishing regular, healthier eating habits – *see* pages 24–7).

2 Instead of flavoured yogurts, add fruit and a drizzle of honey to plain yogurt.

3 Start the day with porridge oats or eggs rather than a ready-to-eat or instant cereal.

4 Bring a packed lunch to work.

5 Cook up a large batch of a simple tomato or vegetable-based pasta sauce and freeze in individual portions (try the Chickpea and Tomato Sauce on page 97).

6 Eat fresh or poached fruit with Greek yogurt instead of fruit pies and crumbles.

7 Carry plain or salted nuts or dried or fresh fruit in your bag or car instead of grabbing UPF snacks on the go.

8 Opt for a sourdough loaf – it's less likely to contain preservatives than most supermarket loaves, even when sliced and packaged.

9 In coffee shops, choose a flat white, cappuccino or latte with dairy milk but no syrups.

10 Dip bread in extra virgin olive oil or use a little bit of butter instead of a margarine spread.

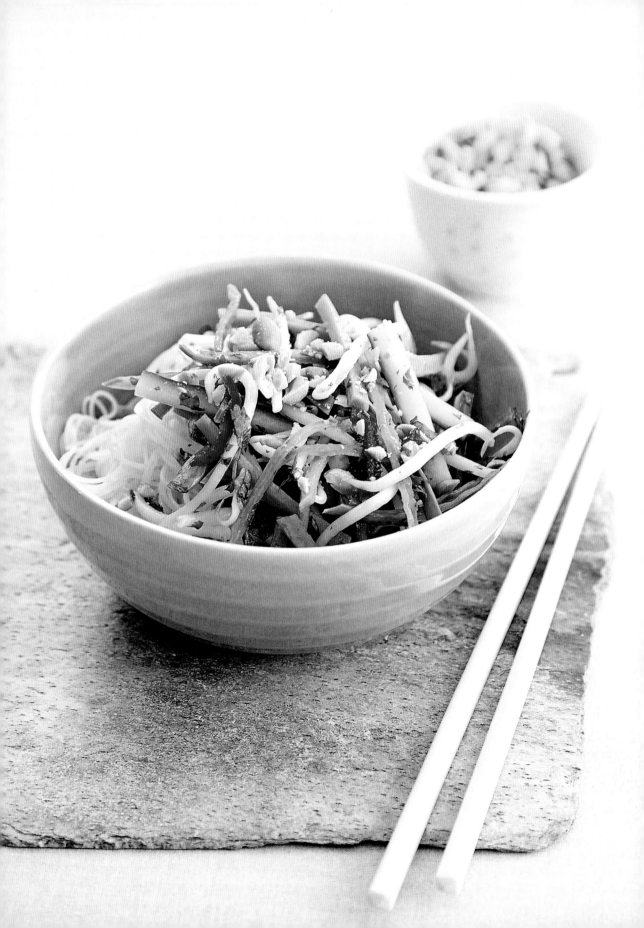

Common sense around UPFs

Although this book is all about helping you to cut out ultra-processed foods, it's true to say that not every food in this group needs to be avoided at all costs. In fact, some foods with overall good nutritional value only stray into UPF territory because of innocuous ingredients such as added fibre extracts (chicory extract, inulin, etc.), whey proteins, soy lecithin and thickening starches. For example, baked beans, tomato pasta sauces, yeast extract, wholemeal bread, almond milk and lower sugar wholegrain cereal all count as UPFs but are far healthier than sweets, cakes and fizzy drinks.

Some chemical-sounding ingredients are also not as worrying as they sound and have more common names outside the context of a food label. For example, plain old baking powder can appear as disodium diphosphate and sodium bicarbonate on a label, while vitamin C can be listed as ascorbic acid. This means that some common sense is needed in following a low UPF diet.

A low UPF diet is healthy, but trying to cut out every single UPF food isn't necessary or helpful. Instead, aim to keep your UPF intake to no more than 20 per cent of your diet. And when you do eat UPFs, choose the healthier ones. If you're wavering as to whether a UPF should be on your shopping list or not, look at the checklist below. On balance it's fine from a health perspective to put food in your basket if it ticks two or more of these four criteria.

- At least 1 g (⁷⁄₂₀₀ oz) of fibre to every 10 g (³⁄₈ oz) of carbohydrate
- Less than 5 g (¼ oz) of sugar per 100 g (3½ oz)
- Less than 1.5 g (¹⁄₂₀ oz) saturated fat per 100 g (3½ oz)
- Less than 0.3 g (¹⁄₁₀₀ oz) salt per 100 g (3½ oz)

It's worth pointing out that cooking everything from scratch doesn't necessarily mean your meals will be nutritionally sound. For example, butter (minimally processed) contains much higher levels of saturated fat than a light spread (ultra-processed). And calories can be high in unprocessed foods such as nuts, cream, avocados, smoked salmon and bacon. The bottom line? To be healthy and reduce your risk of disease you'll still need to keep a watch on saturated fat, sugar, salt and alcohol. If you're trying to keep your weight in check, you'll need to keep an eye on portion sizes and calories too.

A note on our UPF-free recipes

The grey areas that exist around the definition of ultra-processed food means that you'll need to assess your own level of tolerance for specific foods or ingredients. For the recipes in this book we've taken a middle-of-the-road approach, leaving in a handful of foods or ingredients that could, under a very strict interpretation, be regarded as UPF. Usually this is to cut extra hours in the kitchen and to ensure great tasting, fail-safe results.

For clarity, over the page are the 'grey' area ingredients and the stance we have taken on them both in the weekly meal plans and recipes that follow.

Oils

Vegetable oils, including olive oil, are officially in NOVA category 2, i.e. processed culinary ingredients extracted from natural foods or from nature. However, there's an argument that most supermarket vegetable oils are actually UPF because they are extracted with chemical solvent before being refined, bleached and deodorised.

We've largely used extra virgin olive oil in the recipes that follow to get around these issues as it is cold pressed and unrefined. But where a more neutral taste is needed, we've included other oils.

Overall, it's about balance and while over-consuming refined seed oils such as sunflower, rapeseed and groundnut isn't a good idea, neither is there any good evidence that these unsaturated oils harm health, even when highly refined. Organic, cold pressed rapeseed or sunflower oil are good options for our recipes that require vegetable oil if you still have concerns.

Bread

Bread is processed (NOVA category 3) when it's made slowly using a traditional bakery process, but UPF (NOVA category 4) when mass produced. However, though it's fabulous to pick up fresh bakery bread if you can afford it and it's available, many supermarket breads can be just fine too.

The least UPF supermarket choices are seeded wholemeal and sourdough, and you can compare ingredients to check for unwanted preservatives etc. Alternately make your own bread using the recipes on pages 150 and 156.

Dried yeast

Dried yeast and fast-action dried yeast – even the organic versions – require an emulsifier (sorbitan monostearate) to be shelf stable. We've used dried yeast in our recipes, but if you want to use fresh yeast you can. You'll need three times as much fresh yeast as fast-action dried yeast and twice as much fresh yeast as dried yeast. You should also leave more time to prove.

Self-raising flour and raising agents

Popular store cupboard raising agents such as bicarbonate of soda, cream of tartar and baking powder are chemical additives that could technically be construed as UPF. However, they have a long history of traditional use and home baking is impossible without them, so we have allowed these and self-raising flour (which contains them) in our recipes.

Cocoa powder

Cocoa powder comes in two forms: alkalized (sometimes known as 'dutched') and non-alkalized. You'll see acidity regulators such as potassium carbonate on the label of alkalized cocoa powder, and it will be darker and less bitter. Organic cocoa can be alkalized too. The simplest way to avoid this additive is to look for cacao powder, which is almost always non-alkalized.

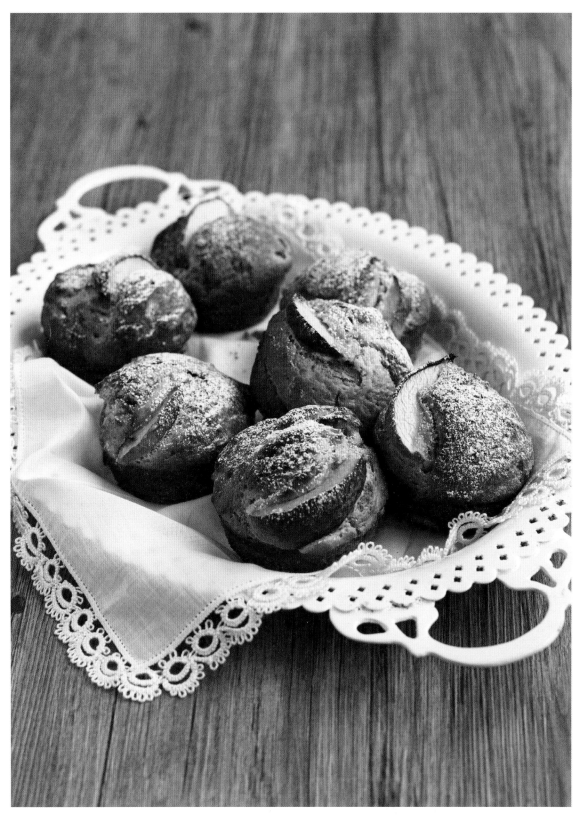

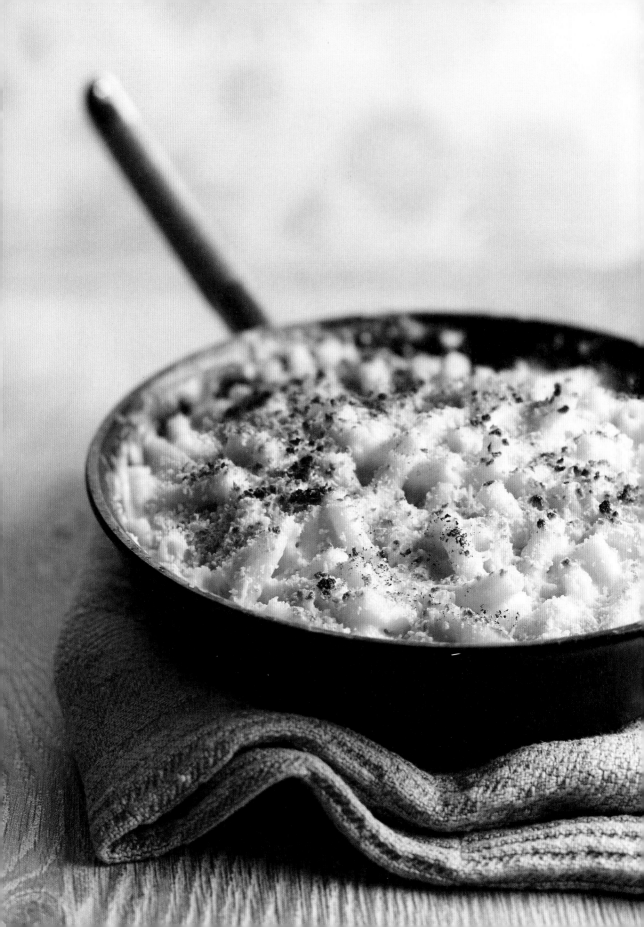

Chocolate

The NOVA classification system categorizes chocolate confectionery as a UPF (category 4), but many bars of dark chocolate will fall into category 3. For a non-UPF option with the highest level of anti-inflammatory plant chemicals, look for an ingredients list comprising only cocoa (cocoa mass), cocoa butter, sugar and vanilla. This will usually be a bar with 70 per cent or more cocoa solids.

Raisins and sultanas

Raisins and sultanas are included in a few of the recipes in this book. They often have a vegetable oil coating to keep them from sticking together so if is this a concern for you, look for organic varieties where the vegetable oil used will likely be unrefined, or missing completely.

Stock

Many forms of shop-bought stock, such as cubes and pots, tend to be UPF. Where stock occurs in our recipes, it would be great if you could make your own. However, there are shop-bought versions that are not so ultra-processed. It's worth comparing labels but supermarket brands often use less UPF ingredients than big brands. You'll also find fewer additives in organic stock and liquid stock (sold in volumes of 500 ml/18 fl oz or more).

Endnotes

1: 'Position statement on the concept of ultra-processed foods (UPF)', British Nutrition Foundation, http://www.nutrition.org.uk/news/2023/position-statement-on-the-concept-of-ultra-processed-foods-upf, April 2023 [accessed 15 February 2024]

2: Southey, Flora, 'Consumers don't know what "ultra-processed" food is, but know they don't want it', FoodNavigator, http://www.foodnavigator.com/Article/2023/04/27/consumers-don-t-know-what-ultra-processed-food-is-but-know-they-don-t-want-it, 27 April 2023 [accessed 15 February 2024]

3: 'Food, Nutrition & Fitness I: The Digestion Journey Begins with Food Choices', http://ecuphysicians.ecu.edu/wp-content/pv-uploads/sites/78/2021/07/NOVA-Classification-Reference-Sheet.pdf, compiled in 2018 by EduChange with guidance from NUPENS, São Paolo [accessed 15 February 2024]

4: Srour, B.; Fezeu, L.K.; Kesse-Guyot, E.; Allès, B.; Méjean, C.; Andrianasolo, R.M.; et al. 'Ultra-processed food intake and risk of cardiovascular disease: prospective cohort study (NutriNet-Santé)', BMJ (2019). https://www.bmj.com/content/365/bmj.l1451 [accessed 16 February 2024]

5: Qu, Y.; Hu, W.; Xing, C.; Yuan, L.; Huang, J. 'Ultra-processed food consumption and cardiovascular events risk', European Heart Journal (2023). https://academic.oup.com/eurheartj/article/44/Supplement_2/ehad655.2389/7391188 [accessed 16 February 2024]

6: Pant, A.; Gribbin, S.; Machado, P.; et al. 'Ultra-processed foods and incident cardiovascular disease and hypertension in middle-aged women', European Journal of Nutrition (2023). https://link.springer.com/article/10.1007/s00394-023-03297-4#citeas [accessed 16 February 2024]

7: Chang, Kiara, Gunter, Marc J., Rauber, Fernanda, Levy, Renata B., Huybrechts, Inge, Kliemann, Nathalie, et al., 'Ultra-processed food consumption, cancer risk and cancer mortality: a large-scale prospective analysis within the UK Biobank', The Lancet, http://www.thelancet.com/journals/eclinm/article/PIIS2589-5370(23)00017-2/fulltext, 31 January 2023 [accessed 15 February 2024]

8: Srour, Bernard, Fezeu, Léopold K., Kesse-Guyot, Emmanuelle, et al., 'Ultraprocessed Food Consumption and Risk of Type 2 Diabetes Among Participants of the NutriNet-Santé Prospective Cohort', JAMA Internal Medicine, http://jamanetwork.com/journals/jamainternalmedicine/article-abstract/2757497, 16 December 2019 [accessed 15 February 2024]

9: Samuthpongtorn, C.; Nguyen, L.H.; Okereke, O.I.; et al. 'Consumption of Ultraprocessed Food and Risk of Depression', JAMA Network Open (2023). https://jamanetwork.com/journals/jamanetworkopen/fullarticle/2809727 [accessed 16 February 2024]

10: Hall, K.D.; Ayuketah, A.; Brychta, R.; Cai, H.; Cassimatis, T.; Chen, K.Y.; Chung, S.T.; Costa, E.; Courville, A.; Darcey, V.; Fletcher, L.A.; Forde, C.G.; Gharib, A.M.; Guo, J.; Howard, R.; Joseph, P.V.; McGehee, S.; Ouwerkerk, R.; Raisinger, K.; Rozga, I.; Stagliano, M.; Walter, M.; Walter, P.J.; Yang, S.; Zhou, M. 'Ultra-Processed Diets Cause Excess Calorie Intake and Weight Gain: An Inpatient Randomized Controlled Trial of Ad Libitum Food Intake', Cell Metabolism (2019). https://pubmed.ncbi.nlm.nih.gov/31105044/ [accessed 16 February 2024]

Sauces and Dressings

Tomato ketchup

Serves 10–15

400 g (14 oz) can chopped tomatoes
2 tablespoons maple syrup
1 tablespoon soft brown sugar
3 tablespoons red wine vinegar

Place all the ingredients into a small, heavy-based frying pan and bring to the boil. Reduce the heat and simmer gently for 5–7 minutes, uncovered, stirring occasionally until the sauce is thick and pulpy. Whizz in a food processor or blender until smooth, then place in a jar and cool. Store in a refrigerator for up to 2 weeks.

Mayonnaise

Serves 6–8

2 egg yolks
2 teaspoons Dijon mustard (see tip, page 100)
1–2 tablespoons white wine vinegar
250 ml (8 fl oz) extra virgin olive oil
salt and pepper

Put the egg yolks, mustard, 1 tablespoon vinegar and a little salt and pepper into a large bowl and whisk lightly with a balloon whisk to combine. Whisking continuously, start adding the olive oil, a few drops at a time, until the sauce starts to thicken.

Gradually add the remaining oil in a very thin, steady stream until the mayonnaise is thick and glossy. Don't add the oil too quickly or the mayonnaise might start to separate. If this happens, try whisking in 1 tablespoon warm water. If the mixture curdles completely, whisk another egg yolk in a separate bowl and gradually whisk it into the curdled sauce.

Check the seasoning, adding a little more vinegar if the sauce tastes bland. Mayonnaise can be kept, covered, in the refrigerator for up to 2 days.

Vinaigrette

Serves 4–6

1 teaspoon caster sugar
pinch of mustard powder
2 tablespoons wine vinegar
4–6 tablespoons extra virgin olive oil
salt and pepper

Put the sugar, mustard powder and vinegar into a small bowl and whisk lightly with a balloon whisk to combine. Add the oil, season to taste with salt and pepper and whisk together thoroughly. Alternatively, put the ingredients in a screw-top jar, replace the lid and shake well.

French dressing

Serves 6–8

½ small onion
6 tablespoons extra virgin olive oil
2 tablespoons wine vinegar
½ teaspoon Dijon mustard (see tip, page 100)
½ tablespoon caster sugar
pinch of ground coriander
3 tablespoons chopped parsley
salt and pepper

Grate the onion and put into a small bowl with the remaining ingredients. Whisk lightly with a balloon whisk until thickened. Season to taste with salt and pepper. Alternatively, put the ingredients, including the grated onion, in a screw-top jar, replace the lid and shake well.

Meal Plans

Here you will find four weekly meal plans to get you started on your journey to quit UPFs for good. Remember to add a portion of fresh vegetables or salad to every main meal.

	Week One			
	Breakfast	**Lunch**	**Dinner**	**Snacks**
Monday	Poached eggs on sourdough toast; glass of pure fruit juice	**Classic Minestrone** (*see* page 57) with **Warm Seedy Rolls** (*see* page 155)	Pea and Mint Risotto (*see* page 92)	Cheese and fruit
Tuesday	**Maple-glazed Granola with Fruit** (*see* page 33)	Vietnamese-style Noodle Salad (*see* page 66)	Chicken breast wrapped in Parma ham, served with buttered new potatoes and vegetables	Unsalted nuts
Wednesday	Sourdough toast topped with full-fat cream cheese and smoked salmon; bowl of berries	**Classic Minestrone** (*see* page 57) with **Warm Seedy Rolls** (*see* page 155)	Grilled salmon, served with stir-fried vegetables and rice	**Peach and Brown Sugar Muffin** (*see* page 164); apple
Thursday	Scrambled eggs with stir-fried mushrooms on toasted bread	Baked potato topped with hummus (additive-free or homemade)	**Moroccan-inspired Vegetable Stew** (*see* page 98)	Olives and feta cubes
Friday	Smashed avocado on sourdough toast, topped with a poached egg	Canned sardines in brine on toasted bread, served with cherry tomatoes	**Frying Pan Macaroni Cheese** (*see* page 94)	Unsalted nuts
Saturday	**Breakfast Banana Split** (*see* page 37)	**Summer Vegetable Tortiglioni with Basil Vinaigrette** (*see* page 70)	**Yellow Chicken Drumstick Curry** (*see* page 110)	**Peach and Brown Sugar Muffin** (*see* page 164); mango
Sunday	**Blueberry Pancakes** (*see* page 42)	**Butter Bean, Tomato and Feta Salad** (*see* page 61)	**Linguine with Chickpea and Tomato Sauce** (*see* page 97)	Unsalted nuts

Week Two

	Breakfast	Lunch	Dinner	Snacks
Monday	Maple-glazed Granola with Fruit (see page 33)	Grilled cheese (grated Cheddar) on sourdough toast, served with cherry tomatoes	Pea and Mint Risotto (see page 92)	Slice of Banana and Pecan Loaf (see page 160)
Tuesday	Scrambled eggs with chopped tomato on toasted bread	Roasted Butternut, Sage and Cashew Soup (see page 62) with Mixed Seed Soda Bread (see page 156)	Stir-fry made with chicken breast, any colourful vegetables, wholewheat noodles and organic tamari soy sauce	Few squares of dark chocolate; apple
Wednesday	Sourdough toast topped with full-fat cream cheese and smoked salmon; bowl of berries	Baked potato topped with sour cream, chives and cold cooked chicken; apple	Baked salmon, served with stir-fried vegetables and rice	Slice of Banana and Pecan Loaf (see page 160)
Thursday	Poached or fried egg, grilled bacon and grilled tomato, served with toasted bread	Roasted Butternut, Sage and Cashew Soup (see page 62) with Mixed Seed Soda Bread (see page 156)	Spicy Turkey Burgers with Red Pepper Salsa (see page 113)	Unsalted nuts
Friday	Porridge with milk, topped with almond butter, blueberries and a drizzle of maple syrup	Sandwich made with Mixed Seed Soda Bread (see page 156), filled with brie and sliced grapes; mango	Classic Bolognese (see page 121)	Popcorn with Chilli Oil (see page 171)
Saturday	Wholemeal Cheese and Bacon Breakfast Muffin (see page 45); glass of pure orange juice	Chicken, Apricot and Almond Salad (see page 74)	Keralan-style Fish Curry (see page 104)	Jerusalem Artichoke Crisps with Sage Salt (see page 172)
Sunday	Moroccan-style Baked Eggs (see page 50)	Chicken and Vegetable Satay (see page 77)	Beef and Lentil Chilli (see page 122)	Potato Skins with Guacamole (see page 179)

Week Three

	Breakfast	Lunch	Dinner	Snacks
Monday	**Toasted Muesli with Coconut Chips** (*see page 38*), served with natural yogurt; glass of pure orange juice	**Roasted Tomato Soup** (*see page 73*) with **Warm Seedy Rolls** (*see page 155*)	**Chargrilled Halloumi with Roasted Olives and Salad** (*see page 91*)	Plain Greek yogurt and berries
Tuesday	**Wholemeal Cheese and Bacon Breakfast Muffin** (*see page 45*); banana	**Roasted Chickpeas with Spinach** (*see page 69*)	Grilled salmon, served with long-stem broccoli and homemade oven chips (just potatoes and vegetable oil)	Few squares of dark chocolate; apple
Wednesday	Smashed avocado on sourdough toast, served with two slices of back bacon	**Roasted Tomato Soup** (*see page 73*) with **Warm Seedy Rolls** (*see page 155*)	**Chicken and Spinach Stew** (*see page 108*)	Unsalted nuts
Thursday	Homemade breakfast smoothie (1 big handful of frozen dark cherries, 1 heaped tsp cocoa powder, 1 tbsp almond butter, 1 small handful of spinach and 150ml/5fl oz milk)	**Chicken, Apricot and Almond Salad** (*see page 74*)	Chicken breast wrapped in Parma ham, served with buttered new potatoes and vegetables	Celery or carrot sticks with hummus (additive-free or homemade)
Friday	Shredded wheat, served with milk, chopped banana and chopped hazelnuts	Grilled cheese (grated Cheddar) on sourdough toast, served with cherry tomatoes	**Easy Fish Pie with Crunchy Potato Topping** (*see page 103*)	Olives and feta cubes
Saturday	**Chocolate Porridge with Berries** (*see page 34*)	**Greek Salad** (*see page 65*)	Steak, served with homemade oven chips (just potatoes and vegetable oil) and a salad of rocket and Parmesan flakes tossed in balsamic vinegar and extra virgin olive oil	Unsalted nuts
Sunday	**Breakfast Banana Split** (*see page 37*)	**Warm Potato and Mackerel Salad** (*see page 78*)	**Lasagne** (*see page 125*)	**Cheese and Chive Crisps** (*see page 175*)

Week Four

	Breakfast	Lunch	Dinner	Snacks
Monday	Chocolate and Raisin Porridge Bar (*see* page 34); banana	Vietnamese-style Noodle Salad (*see* page 66)	**Sweet and Sour Pork** (*see* page 117)	Unsalted nuts
Tuesday	**Toasted Muesli with Coconut Chips** (*see* page 38), served with milk and blueberries	Baked potato topped with hummus (additive-free or homemade); orange	Stir-fry made with king prawns, any colourful vegetables, wholewheat noodles and organic tamari soy sauce	Celery or carrot sticks with hummus (additive-free or homemade)
Wednesday	Homemade breakfast smoothie (½ banana, 1 big handful of strawberries, 1 tbsp almond butter and 150ml/5fl oz milk)	Canned sardines in brine on toasted bread, served with chopped cucumber and celery	**Cod Fillets with Tomatoes and Salsa Verde** (*see* page 100)	Few squares of dark chocolate; apple
Thursday	**Potato and Sweetcorn Hash with Frazzled Eggs** (*see* page 41)	**Chicken and Aduki Bean Salad** (*see* page 81)	**King Prawn and Courgette Linguine** (*see* page 107)	Unsalted nuts
Friday	**Breakfast Banana Split** (*see* page 37)	**Butternut Squash and Ricotta Frittata** (*see* page 85)	Grilled salmon, served with stir-fried vegetables and rice	Cheese and fruit
Saturday	Moroccan-style Baked Eggs (*see* page 50); glass of pure orange juice	Chicken and Tarragon Pesto Penne (*see* page 82)	Fiorentina Pizza (*see* page 88)	**Popcorn with Chilli Oil** (*see* page 171)
Sunday	**Blueberry Pancakes** (*see* page 42)	**Fresh Herb Pasta Salad** (*see* page 58)	**Mediterranean Roast Lamb** (*see* page 118)	Plain Greek yogurt and berries

Breakfasts

French Toast

Serves 4

2 eggs, beaten
1 teaspoon vanilla extract (optional)
100 ml (3½ fl oz) milk
1 tablespoon caster sugar, plus extra
    for sprinkling
½ teaspoon ground cinnamon
4 thick slices of sourdough bread
25 g (1 oz) butter

1 Whisk the eggs with the vanilla extract (if using), milk, sugar and cinnamon in a shallow dish. Place the slices of bread in the mixture, turning to coat both sides so that they absorb the liquid.

2 Heat the butter in a nonstick frying pan. Use a palette knife or fish slice to transfer the soaked bread to the hot pan and fry for 2 minutes on each side until golden.

3 Cut the toasts in half diagonally, sprinkle with a little caster sugar and serve immediately.

Apple and Raspberry Sauce

Heat 25 g (1 oz) butter in a frying pan, add 6 peeled, cored and sliced eating apples and fry for 2–3 minutes. Sprinkle over 1 tablespoon light soft brown sugar, ½ teaspoon ground cinnamon and 125 g (4 oz) raspberries and cook gently for 1–2 minutes. Pour over the French toast and sprinkle with extra caster sugar.

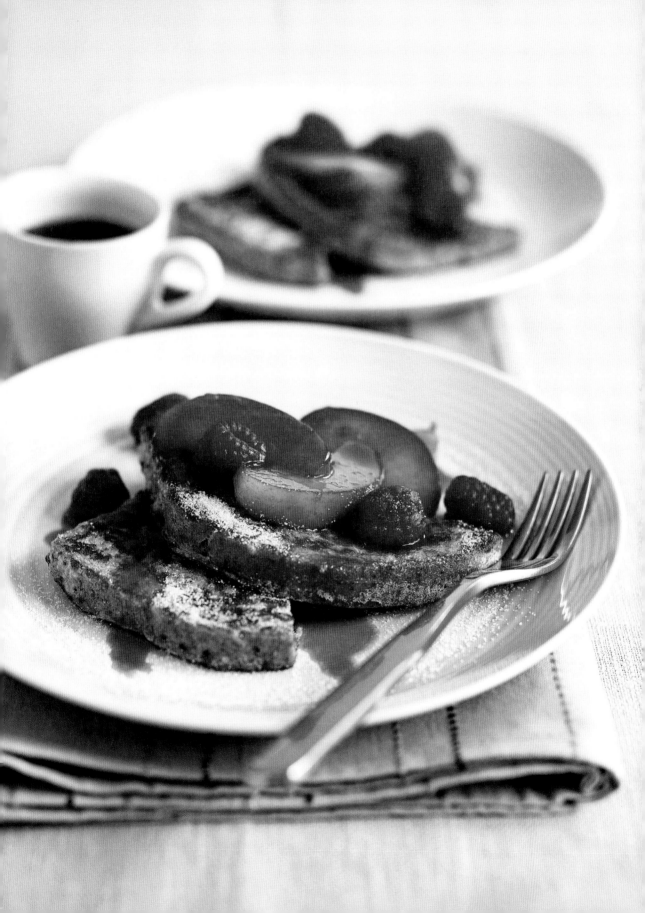

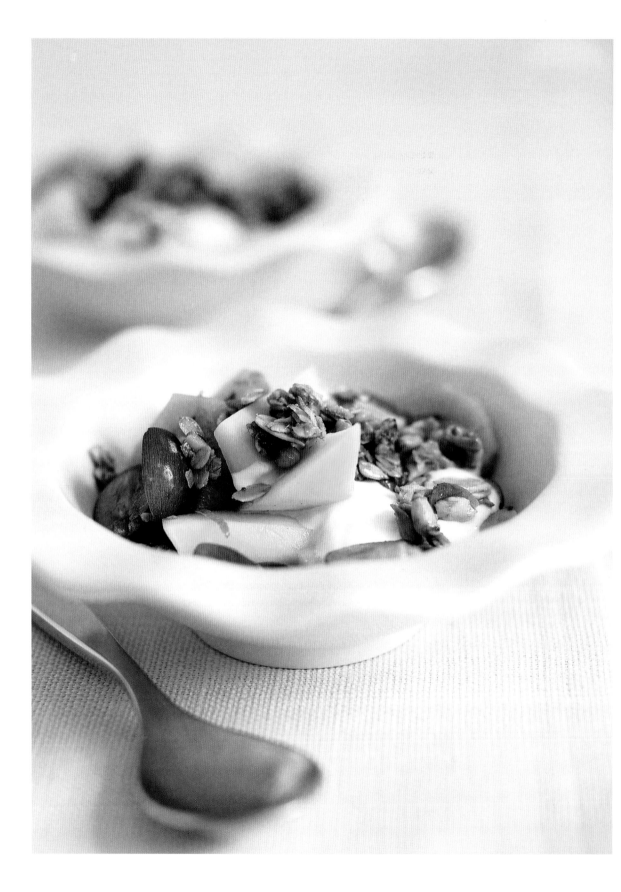

Maple-glazed Granola with Fruit

Serves 6

2 tablespoons extra virgin olive oil
2 tablespoons maple syrup
40 g (1½ oz) flaked almonds
40 g (1½ oz) pine nuts
25 g (1 oz) sunflower seeds
25 g (1 oz) porridge oats
375 ml (12 fl oz) low-fat natural
    yogurt, to serve

Fruit salad
1 mango, stoned, peeled and sliced
2 kiwifruit, peeled and sliced
1 small bunch of red seedless
    grapes, halved
grated rind and juice of
    1 unwaxed lime

1 Heat the oil in a flameproof frying pan with a metal handle, add the maple syrup and the nuts, seeds and oats and toss together.

2 Transfer the pan to a preheated oven, 180°C (350°F), Gas Mark 4, and cook for 5–8 minutes, stirring once and moving the brown edges to the centre, until the granola mixture is evenly toasted.

3 Leave the mixture to cool, then pack it into a storage jar, seal, label and consume within 10 days.

4 Make the fruit salad just before serving. Mix the fruits with the lime rind and juice, spoon the mixture into 6 dishes and top with spoonfuls of natural yogurt and granola.

Berry Compote
Place 150 g (5 oz) each of raspberries, blackberries and blueberries in a pan with the grated rind and juice of 1 unwaxed lemon. Heat gently until the fruit has softened and the blueberries burst, then sweeten with 1 teaspoon clear honey. Serve with the granola and yogurt, as above, instead of the fruit salad.

Chocolate Porridge with Berries

Serves 2

600 ml (1 pint) milk
100 g (3½ oz) porridge oats
3 tablespoons cocoa or cacao powder,
    plus extra for dusting (optional)
4 tablespoons soft brown sugar
75 g (3 oz) mixed berries
2 tablespoons maple syrup

1 Place the milk in a heavy-based saucepan with the oats and bring to the boil. Add the cocoa or cacao powder and sugar, then reduce the heat and simmer for 6–7 minutes, stirring occasionally, until the oats have swollen and the porridge has thickened, adding a little water to loosen if necessary.

2 Mix the berries with the maple syrup. Serve the porridge in warmed serving bowls with the berries spooned into the centre. Dust with cocoa or cacao powder, if liked.

Chocolate and Raisin Porridge Bars
Place 300 ml (½ pint) boiling water in a saucepan with 100 g (3½ oz) porridge oats, 50 g (2 oz) raisins, 3 tablespoons cocoa or cacao powder and 4 tablespoons soft brown sugar and bring back to the boil. Reduce the heat to a simmer and stir continuously for about 2–3 minutes until very thick. Transfer to a 20 cm (8 inch) square cake tin and smooth the top. Chill for 20 minutes until solid, then cut into 12 squares or bars to serve (these will keep for up to 3 days refrigerated in an airtight container).

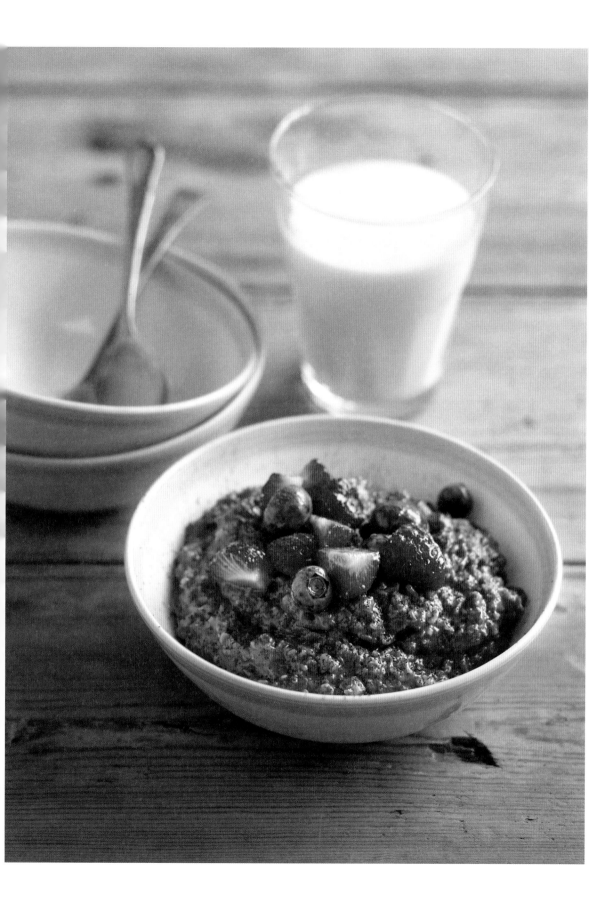

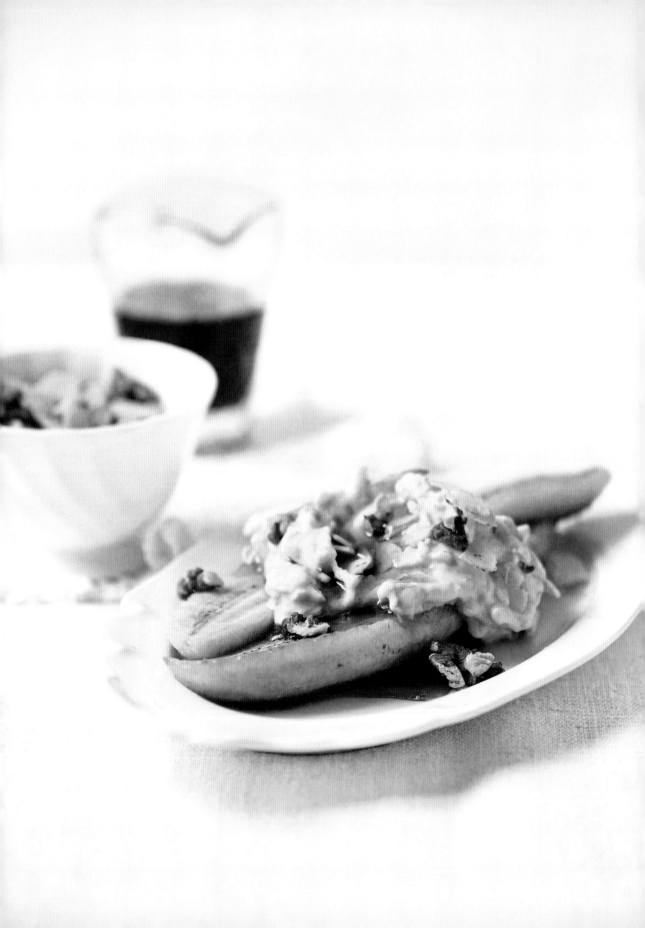

Breakfast Banana Split

Serves 4

50 g (2 oz) unsalted butter
2 tablespoons clear honey
4 bananas, cut in half lengthways
2 dessert apples, grated
300 g (10 oz) Greek yogurt
finely grated rind of
   1 unwaxed orange
50 g (2 oz) walnuts, toasted
2 tablespoons flaked
   almonds, toasted
2–3 tablespoons maple syrup

1 Melt the butter in a frying pan with the honey until it sizzles.

2 Place the bananas in the frying pan, cut side down, and cook for 3–4 minutes, until golden.

3 Meanwhile, mix together the grated apple, yogurt and orange rind.

4 Spoon the bananas onto 4 warmed plates and top with a large dollop of the yogurt mixture.

5 Sprinkle over the nuts, then drizzle with the maple syrup and any juices from the pan to serve.

Banana Buckwheat Pancakes
Place 125 g (4 oz) buckwheat flour in a bowl and whisk in 3 egg yolks, 1 teaspoon clear honey, ¼ teaspoon baking powder and a pinch of ground cinnamon. Slowly whisk in 150 ml (¼ pint) milk. In a grease-free bowl, whisk 3 egg whites until soft peaks form and fold into the batter. Heat 1 tablespoon vegetable oil in a frying pan over a medium heat, add 4 tablespoonfuls of the batter and cook for 2–3 minutes on each side, until golden. Repeat with the remaining batter and keep warm. Meanwhile, in another frying pan melt 50 g (2 oz) butter with 2 tablespoons clear honey, then stir in 3 sliced bananas and cook for 3–4 minutes, until golden. Spoon the honeyed bananas over the pancakes to serve.

Toasted Muesli with Coconut Chips

Serves 8

350 g (11½ oz) rolled oats
75 g (3 oz) organic coconut chips
    or flakes
75 g (3 oz) sunflower seeds
200 g (7 oz) pumpkin seeds
150 g (5 oz) flaked almonds
100 g (3½ oz) hazelnuts
4 tablespoons maple syrup
2 tablespoons vegetable oil
250 g (8 oz) sultanas
75 g (3 oz) dates, roughly chopped

To serve
milk
raspberries

1 Mix together the oats, coconut chips or flakes, sunflower and pumpkin seeds, flaked almonds and hazelnuts in a large bowl.

2 Transfer half of the muesli mixture to a separate bowl. Mix the maple syrup and oil together in a jug, then pour over the remaining half of the muesli and toss really well to lightly coat all the ingredients.

3 Line a large roasting tin with nonstick baking paper, scatter over the syrup-coated muesli and spread out in a single layer. Bake in a preheated oven, 150°C (300°F), Gas Mark 2, for 15–20 minutes, stirring occasionally, until golden and crisp.

4 Leave to cool completely, then toss with the uncooked muesli and the dried fruit. Store in airtight storage jars. Serve with milk and raspberries.

Tip: Some coconut chips have additives, so look for those that are 100 per cent dried coconut (organic versions are more likely to fit the bill).

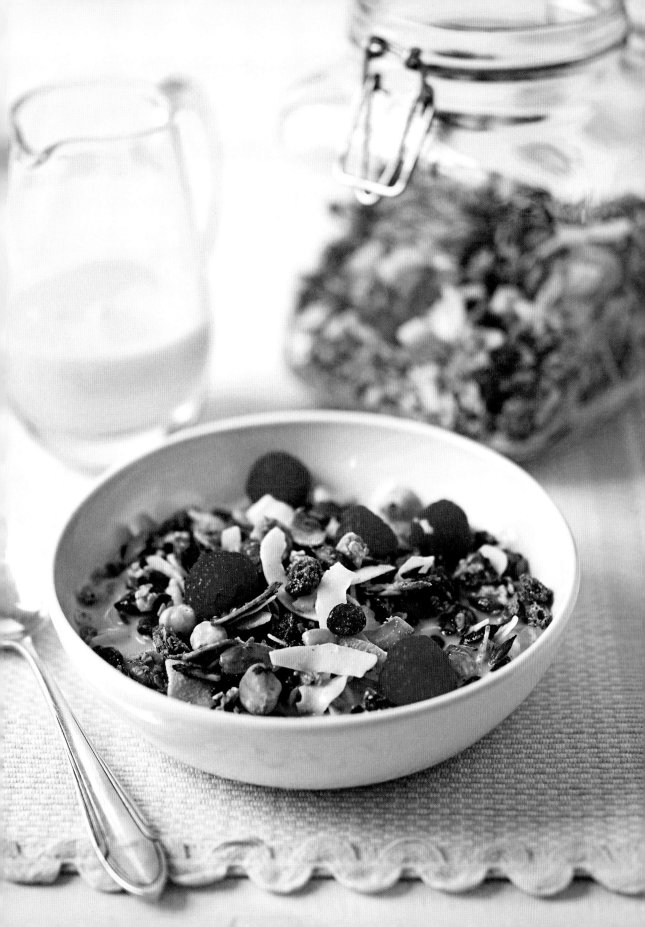

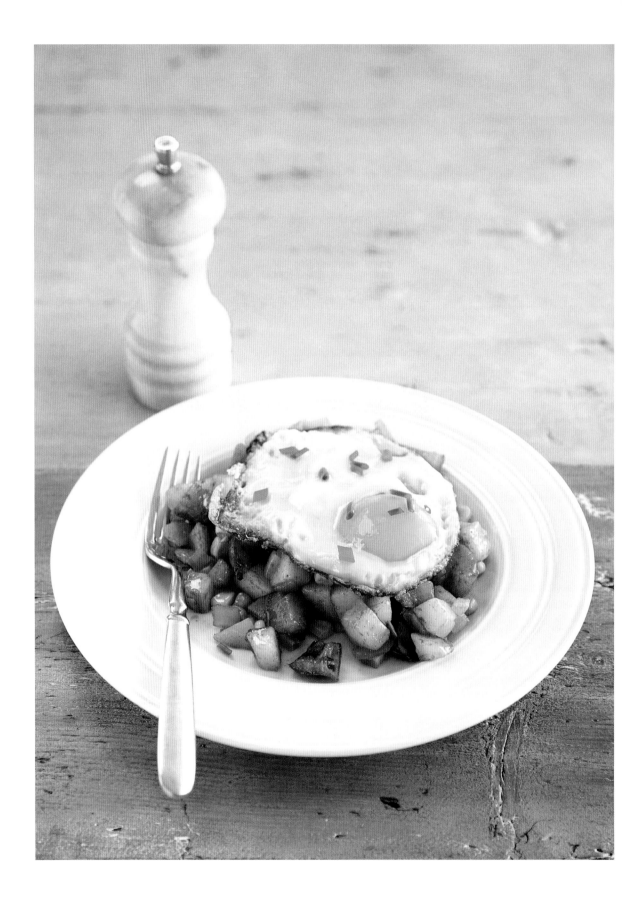

Potato and Sweetcorn Hash with Frazzled Eggs

Serves 4

750 g (1½ lb) large potatoes, peeled and diced
3 tablespoons extra virgin olive oil
1 large onion, finely chopped
1 large green pepper, cored, deseeded and chopped

1 teaspoon smoked paprika
200 g (7 oz) can sweetcorn, drained
4 large eggs
2 tablespoons snipped chives
salt and pepper

1 Put the potatoes in a large saucepan and cover with lightly salted water. Bring to the boil and cook for 12–15 minutes until tender, then drain in a colander.

2 Meanwhile, heat 2 tablespoons of the oil in a large nonstick ovenproof frying pan over a medium heat. Add the onion and green pepper and cook, stirring occasionally, for 7–8 minutes until softened and lightly golden. Add the cooked potatoes, smoked paprika and sweetcorn, season generously with salt and pepper and cook for 3–4 minutes, stirring frequently.

3 Slide the pan under a preheated medium grill, keeping the handle away from the heat, and grill for 2–3 minutes until crispy.

4 While the hash is grilling, heat the remaining oil in a large frying pan then place over a medium heat. Crack the eggs into the pan and fry for 3 minutes until the egg whites are set and crispy.

5 Divide the hash between plates and top each serving with a fried egg. Serve immediately sprinkled with the chives.

Spanish-style Sweetcorn Tortilla
Thinly slice 500 g (1 lb) small potatoes and cook in lightly salted boiling water for 10–12 minutes until tender. Meanwhile, pan-fry 1 finely chopped large onion and 1 large deseeded and chopped green pepper in 1 tablespoon extra virgin olive oil, as above. Add 1 teaspoon smoked paprika and 200 g (7 oz) can sweetcorn, drained, and cook for a further minute. Beat 6 eggs in a bowl and season generously with salt and pepper. Drain the potatoes and stir into the pan with the onions and peppers. Add the eggs, cover loosely and cook for 3–4 minutes, without stirring. Invert the tortilla onto a plate and slide back into the pan for a further 3–4 minutes until firm. Slide onto a board and serve in wedges.

Blueberry Pancakes

Serves 4

250 ml (8 fl oz) milk
2 eggs
100 g (3½ oz) caster sugar
75 g (3 oz) butter, melted, plus extra
    for greasing
1 teaspoon baking powder
pinch of salt
250 g (8 oz) plain flour
100 g (3½ oz) blueberries, plus extra
    to serve
maple syrup or clear honey, to serve

1 Whisk together the milk, eggs, sugar and melted butter in a large bowl. Whisk in the baking powder and salt, add half the flour and whisk well until all the ingredients are incorporated, then whisk in the remaining flour. Stir in the blueberries to mix well.

2 Heat a large, nonstick pan over a medium–high heat. Grease the base of the pan with a little melted butter using kitchen paper. Lower the heat to medium. Spoon in large tablespoons of the batter until the pan is full, allowing a little space between each pancake. Add extra butter for frying if required.

3 Cook for 1–2 minutes on each side or until golden brown, then set aside and keep warm. Continue until all the batter is used.

4 Divide the pancakes between 4 plates that have been warmed in a preheated oven, 150°C (300°F), Gas Mark 2, and drizzle over a little maple syrup or honey. Serve immediately, with extra blueberries.

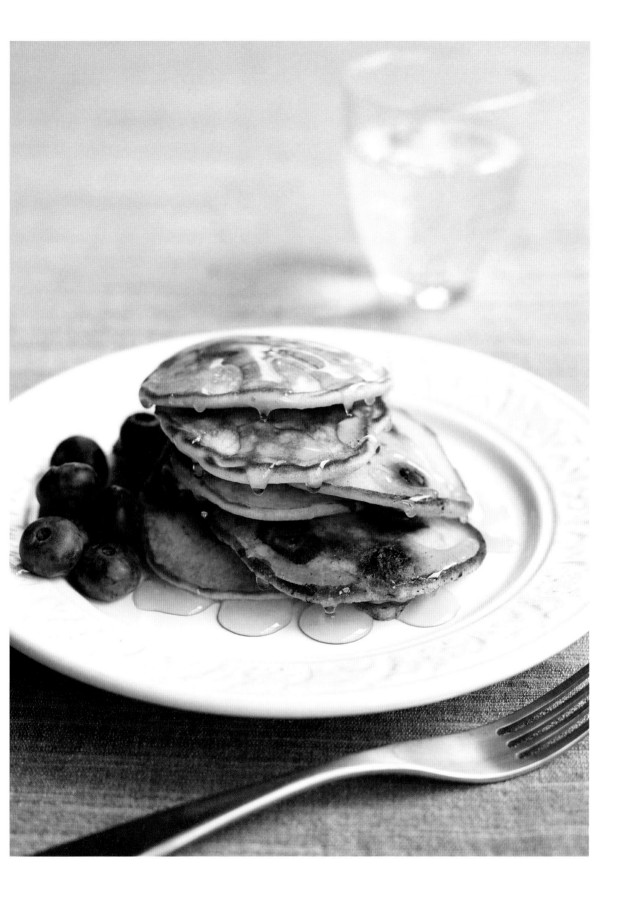

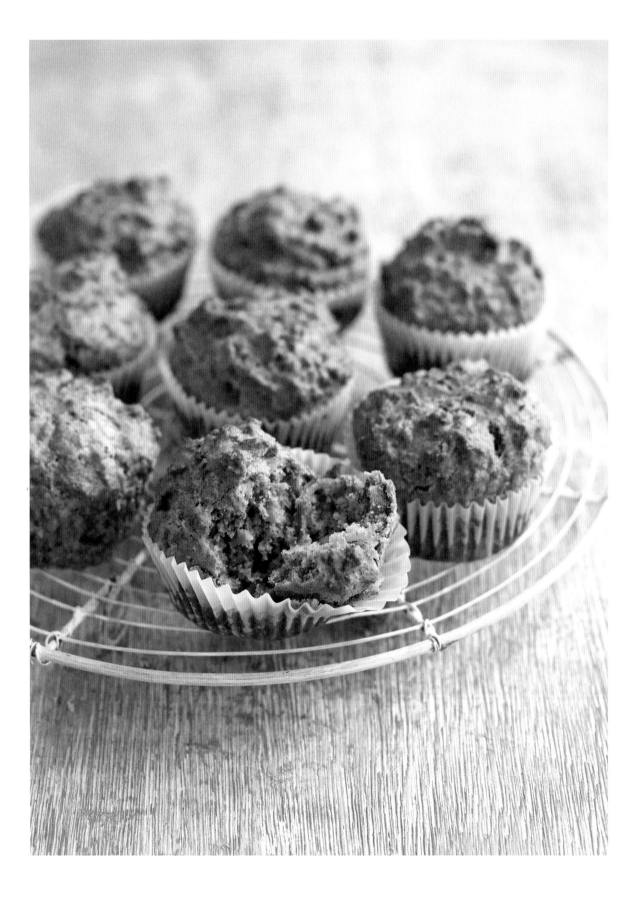

Wholemeal Cheese and Bacon Breakfast Muffins

Makes 12

375 g (12 oz) wholemeal
   self-raising flour
1 teaspoon baking powder
1 teaspoon bicarbonate of soda
2 teaspoons mustard powder
25 g (1 oz) oatbran
125 g (4 oz) Cheddar cheese, grated
50 g (2 oz) cooked bacon pieces,
   chopped
2 eggs
75 ml (3 fl oz) vegetable oil
200 ml (7 fl oz) milk, plus a splash
   (if needed)
salt and pepper

> **Tip:** Bacon is classified as 'processed', not UPF, but it's a good idea to limit how much you eat anyway because of the link between red and processed meat and colorectal cancer.

1   Line a 12-hole muffin tin with 12 paper muffin cases.

2   Sift the flour, baking powder, bicarbonate of soda and mustard powder into a bowl, add the oatbran and then season with a pinch of salt and pepper. Stir in the cheese and bacon pieces.

3   Mix together the egg with the oil and milk in a jug, then pour into the dry ingredients and mix well, adding a little extra milk if the mixture is too dry.

4   Divide the mixture evenly between the paper cases and bake in a preheated oven, 180°C (350°F), Gas Mark 4, for 20–25 minutes until golden and risen.

5   Serve warm if possible, but they are equally delicious cold.

Cheese and Bacon Traybake

Place 250 g (8 oz) self-raising wholemeal flour in a bowl with 1 teaspoon baking powder and 1 teaspoon mustard powder. Mix in 75 g (3 oz) grated Cheddar cheese and 50 g (2 oz) chopped cooked bacon pieces and stir well. Beat 1 egg with 50 ml (2 fl oz) vegetable oil and 50 ml (2 fl oz) milk in a jug, then pour into the dry ingredients and mix well. Pour into a well-greased 18 × 28 cm (7 × 11 inch) ovenproof dish and bake in a preheated oven, 180°C (350°F), Gas Mark 4, for 12–15 minutes until well risen and golden.

Sweetcorn Fritters

Serves 4

200 g (7 oz) self-raising flour
1 egg, beaten
150 ml (¼ pint) milk
200 g (7 oz) sweetcorn (drained,
    if canned, or thawed, if frozen)
1 tablespoon extra virgin olive oil
4 eggs
salt and pepper
snipped chives, to serve

1 Place the flour in a large bowl and whisk in the egg and milk to make a smooth batter.

2 Stir in the sweetcorn and season with salt and pepper.

3 Heat the oil in a frying pan over a medium heat, spoon in tablespoons of the batter (the number of fritters you can make at one time will depend on the size of your pan) and cook for 2–3 minutes on each side, until golden. Repeat with the remaining batter.

4 Meanwhile, poach the eggs in a frying pan of simmering water for 4–5 minutes.

5 Serve a few fritters topped with a poached egg and a sprinkling of chopped chives.

Sweetcorn and Potato Frittata

Cook 675 g (1 lb 5 oz) peeled and sliced potatoes in a large saucepan of boiling water for 2–3 minutes until tender. Drain. Heat 2 tablespoons extra virgin olive oil in a ovenproof frying pan, add 1 sliced onion and 1 deseeded and diced red pepper and cook for 2–3 minutes, then remove with a slotted spoon. Beat 8 eggs in a large bowl and stir in the potato mixture, 400 g (13 oz) sweetcorn and 2 tablespoons chopped parsley and season well with salt and pepper. Heat another tablespoon extra virgin olive oil in the frying pan and gently pour in the egg mixture, moving the ingredients around a little as the egg starts to cook. Continue to cook over a low heat for 12–15 minutes, until the underneath is golden. Sprinkle over 50 g (2 oz) grated Cheddar and place the frying pan under a preheated hot grill for 5–6 minutes, until golden and bubbling. Turn the frittata out onto a board and cut into wedges to serve.

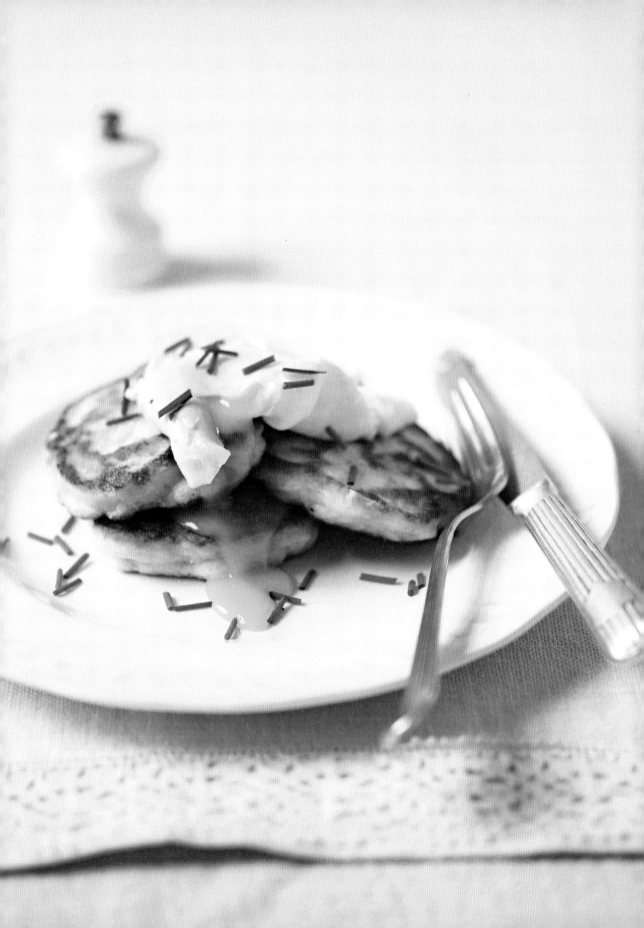

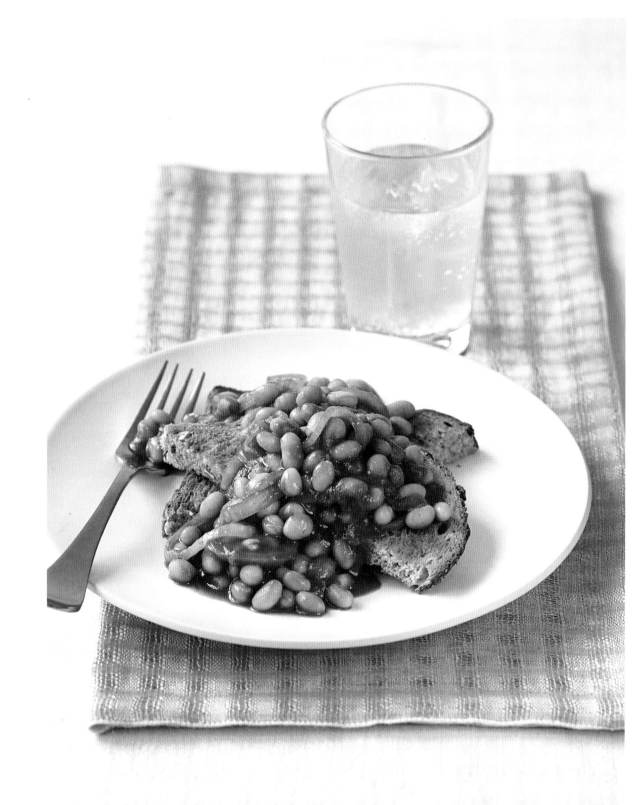

Baked Beans

Serves 4

2 tablespoons extra virgin olive oil
   or vegetable oil
1 onion, thinly sliced
2 garlic cloves, crushed
500 g (1 lb) passata
100 ml (3½ fl oz) hot vegetable stock
   or water
½ teaspoon sugar
2 × 400 g (13 oz) cans haricot beans,
   drained and rinsed
pinch of cayenne (optional)
pinch of ground cinnamon (optional)
salt and pepper
4 slices of sourdough bread or Mixed
   Sead Soda Bread (see page 156),
   toasted, to serve

Tip: Passata is a brilliant source of the antioxidant lycopene. Look for an ingredients list that is just tomatoes or tomatoes and salt.

1 Heat the oil in a heavy-based saucepan and cook the onion gently for 3–4 minutes. Add the garlic and cook for a further 2 minutes, until softened and golden.

2 Add the passata, stock, sugar, beans and spices (if using) and season to taste with salt and pepper. Simmer gently for 12–14 minutes, until rich and thick.

3 Meanwhile, toast the bread until golden and place on 4 plates. Serve the beans spooned over the toast.

Bean Salad

Place 2 × 400 g (13 oz) cans haricot beans, drained and rinsed, in a bowl and add 3 diced tomatoes, 1 crushed garlic clove, 1 finely chopped red onion, 3 tablespoons extra virgin olive oil, a pinch of sugar and 1 tablespoon red wine vinegar. Stir to combine, then spoon into bowls and serve.

Moroccan-style Baked Eggs

Serves 2

½ tablespoon extra virgin olive oil
½ onion, chopped
1 garlic clove, sliced
½ teaspoon ras el hanout
pinch of ground cinnamon
½ teaspoon ground coriander
400 g (13 oz) cherry tomatoes
2 tablespoons chopped coriander
2 eggs
salt and pepper

1 Heat the oil in a frying pan, add the onion and garlic and cook for 6–7 minutes until softened and lightly golden. Stir in the spices and cook, stirring, for a further 1 minute.

2 Add the tomatoes and season well with salt and pepper, then simmer gently for 8–10 minutes.

3 Scatter over 1 tablespoon of the coriander, then divide the tomato mixture between 2 individual ovenproof dishes. Break an egg into each dish.

4 Bake in a preheated oven, 220°C (425°F), Gas Mark 7, for 8–10 minutes until the egg whites are set but the yolks are still slightly runny. Cook for a further 2–3 minutes if you prefer the eggs to be cooked through. Serve scattered with the remaining coriander.

Baked Eggs

Heat 1 tablespoon extra virgin olive oil in a frying pan, add 1 chopped onion and 1 cored, deseeded and chopped red pepper and cook until softened. Add 2 crushed garlic cloves and ½ teaspoon chilli powder and cook, stirring, for a further 1 minute. Stir in a 400 g (13 oz) can chopped tomatoes and simmer gently for 8–10 minutes, then add 1 tablespoon chopped coriander. Divide between 2 individual ovenproof dishes and break an egg into each, then bake as above. Serve with 1 stoned, peeled and sliced avocado, if liked.

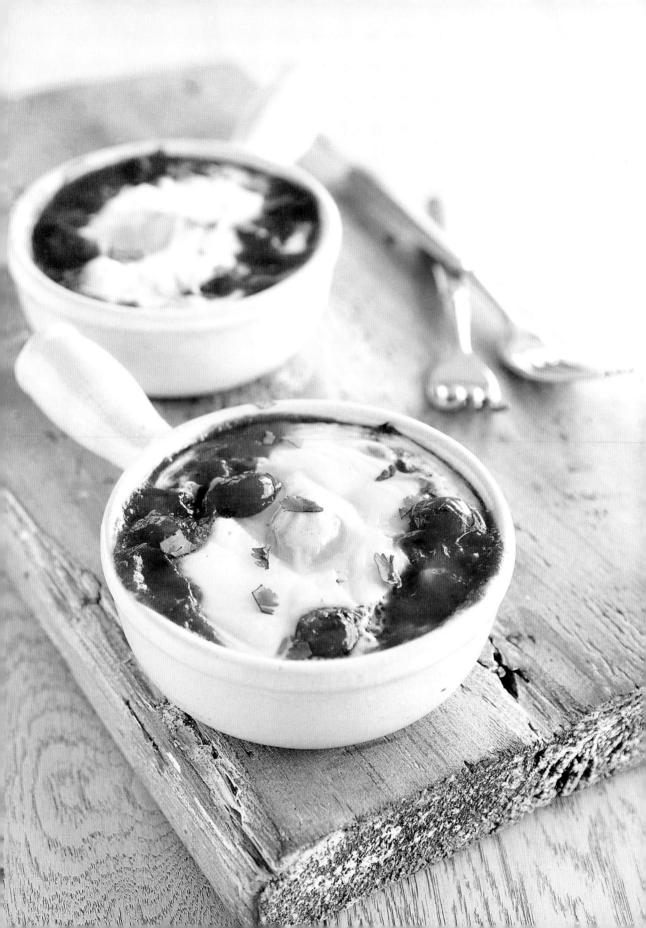

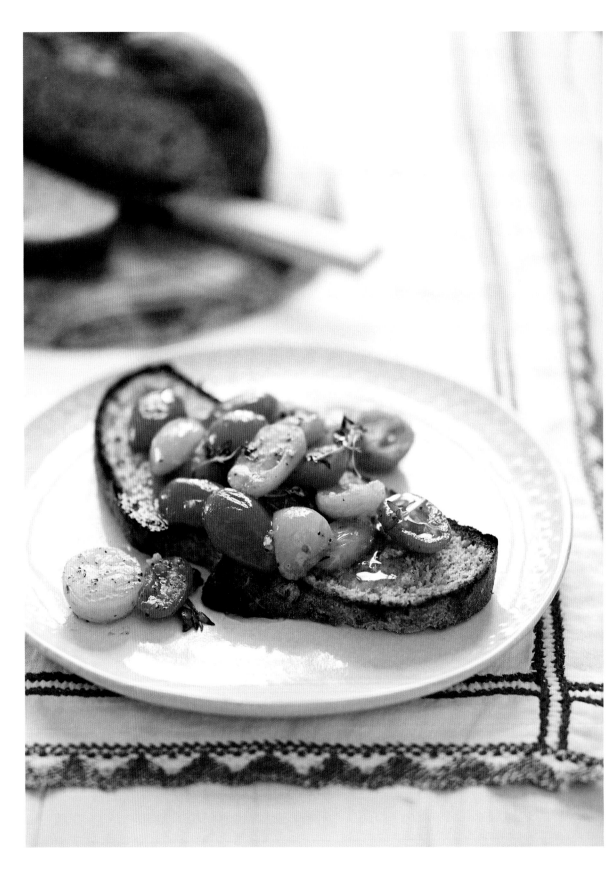

Potato Bread with Tomatoes

Serves 4

375 g (12 oz) potato, peeled and cut into chunks

1 teaspoon fast-action dried yeast (see page 18)

1 teaspoon caster sugar

1 tablespoon extra virgin olive oil, plus extra for oiling

200 g (7 oz) strong white bread flour, plus extra for dusting

100 g (3½ oz) strong wholemeal bread flour

2 tablespoons chopped rosemary

1 tablespoon thyme leaves

salt and pepper

Topping

2 tablespoons extra virgin olive oil

250 g (8 oz) mixed-coloured baby tomatoes, halved

½ teaspoon thyme leaves

½ teaspoon sea salt flakes

1 Cook the potato in a large saucepan of lightly salted boiling water for 15–20 minutes until tender but not flaky. Drain really well, reserving the cooking liquid. Put 6 tablespoons of the cooking liquid into a large bowl and leave to cool until lukewarm. Sprinkle over the yeast, then stir in the sugar and set aside for 10 minutes.

2 Mash the potatoes with the oil, then stir in the yeast mixture and mix well with a wooden spoon. Mix in the flours, herbs and salt and pepper, then turn out on to a lightly floured surface and knead well to incorporate the last of the flour. Knead the dough until soft and pliable, then put in a lightly oiled bowl, cover with clingfilm and leave to rise in a warm place for 1 hour until well risen.

3 Knead the dough on a lightly floured surface, then roughly shape into a round, place on a baking tray and lightly cover with oiled clingfilm. Leave to prove in a warm place for 30 minutes. Score a cross into the dough with a knife and bake in a preheated oven, 220°C (425°F), Gas Mark 7, for 35–40 minutes until well risen and crusty on top. Transfer to a wire rack to cool for 30 minutes.

4 Cut 4 slices of the bread and lightly toast. Meanwhile, heat the oil for the topping in a frying pan, add the tomatoes and cook over a high heat for 2–3 minutes until softened. Stir in the thyme and salt flakes. Serve with the toasted bread, seasoned with pepper.

Sweet Potato and Onion Seed Bread

Prepare the dough as above, using 375 g (12 oz) sweet potato, peeled and chopped, in place of the potato and boiling for 8–10 minutes until just tender, and 2 tablespoons onion seeds instead of the herbs. Bake as above.

Lunches

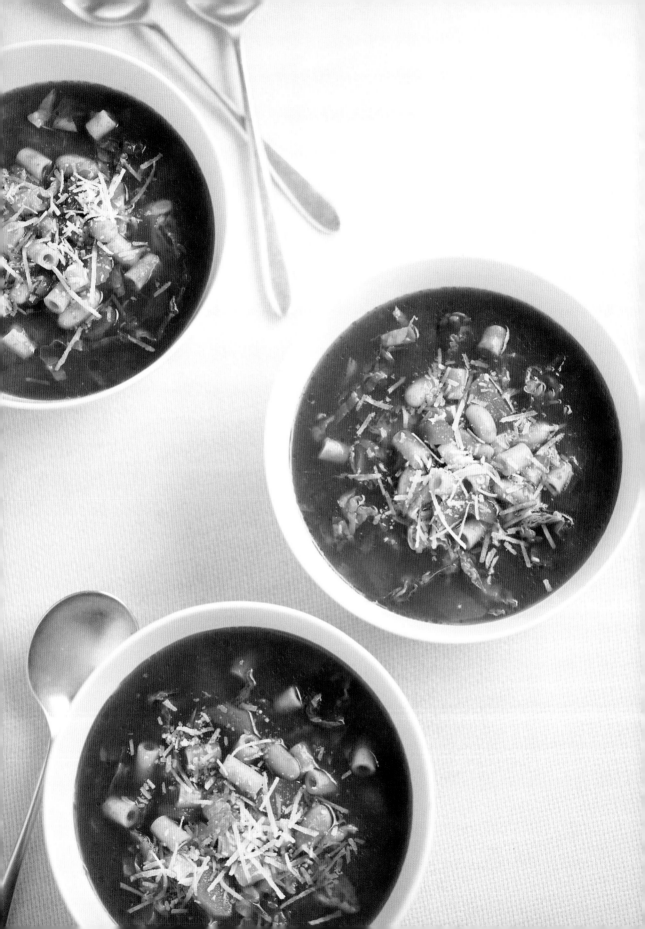

Classic Minestrone

Serves 4

2 tablespoons extra virgin olive oil
1 onion, chopped
1 carrot, peeled and chopped
1 celery stick, chopped
1 teaspoon tomato purée
2 garlic cloves, finely chopped
400 g (13 oz) can chopped tomatoes
750 ml (1¼ pints) hot chicken or
   vegetable stock
2 thyme sprigs, leaves stripped
125 g (4 oz) ditalini pasta
400 g (13 oz) can cannellini beans,
   drained and rinsed
½ head of Savoy cabbage, shredded
salt and pepper
grated Parmesan cheese, to serve

1 Heat the oil in a large saucepan, add the onion, carrot and celery and cook over a low heat for 10 minutes until really soft.

2 Stir in the tomato purée and garlic, then add the tomatoes, stock and thyme and simmer for 10 minutes.

3 Add the pasta and beans to the soup and cook for a further 10 minutes or until the pasta is cooked through. Add the cabbage 5 minutes before the end of the cooking time and cook until tender. Season well.

4 Ladle into serving bowls and serve scattered with the grated Parmesan cheese.

Speedy Springtime Minestrone
Heat 1 tablespoon extra virgin olive oil in a large saucepan, add 1 crushed garlic clove and cook for 30 seconds. Pour over 1 litre (1¾ pints) boiling vegetable stock, then stir in 125 g (4 oz) ditalini pasta and cook for 8 minutes or until cooked through. Add 50 g (2 oz) trimmed green beans and 1 large chopped and deseeded tomato 5 minutes before the end of the cooking time, and 50 g (2 oz) frozen broad beans and 50 g (2 oz) frozen peas 3–4 minutes before the end of the cooking time, cooking until the vegetables are tender. Serve as above.

Fresh Herb Pasta Salad

Serves 4

200 g (7 oz) orzo
5 tablespoons extra virgin olive oil
juice of ½ lemon
2 spring onions, chopped
¼ cucumber, finely chopped
150 g (5 oz) tomatoes, chopped
large handful of flat-leaf
    parsley, chopped
small handful of mint leaves,
    chopped
salt and pepper

1 Cook the orzo in a large saucepan of salted boiling water according to the packet instructions.

2 Drain, then cool under cold running water and drain again.

3 Tip into a serving dish and stir in the oil and lemon juice and season well. Toss through the remaining ingredients and serve.

Simple Herby Pasta

Cook the orzo as above. Drain and return to the pan. Stir in 25 g (1 oz) butter, the chopped herbs as above and a squeeze of lemon juice. Serve immediately.

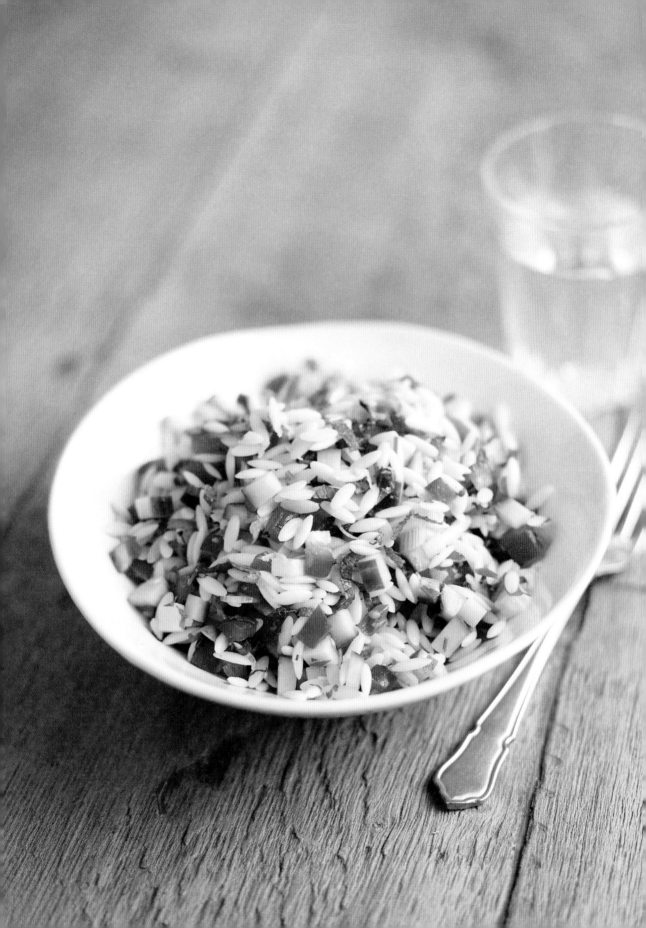

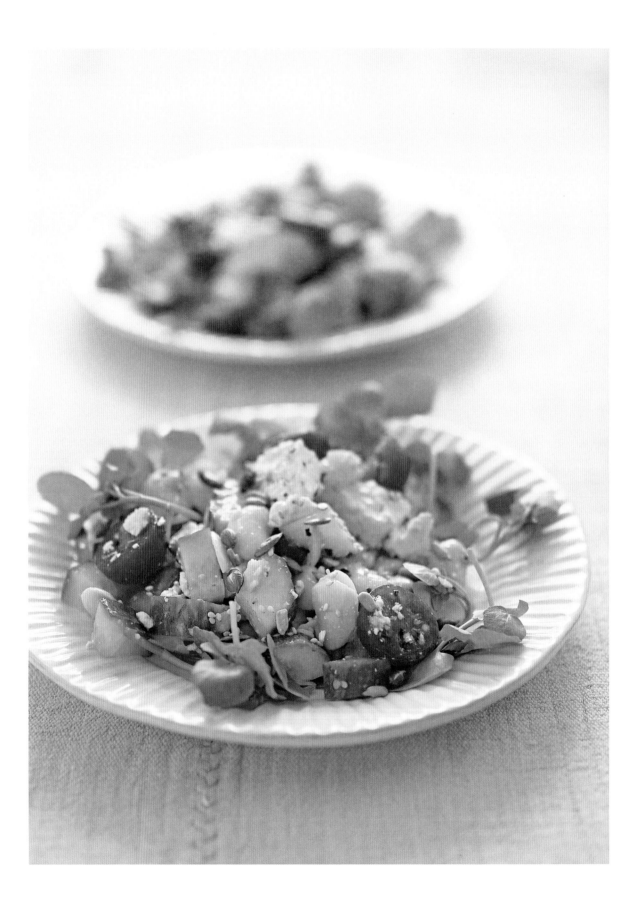

Butter Bean, Tomato and Feta Salad

Serves 4

400 g (13 oz) can butter beans,
    drained and rinsed
18 cherry tomatoes, halved
½ cucumber, chopped
175 g (6 oz) feta cheese, crumbled
juice of 1 lemon
1 teaspoon dried chilli flakes
2 tablespoons extra virgin olive oil
60 g (2½ oz) watercress
2 teaspoons sunflower seeds
1 teaspoon pumpkin seeds
½ teaspoon sesame seeds

1 Place the butter beans, cherry tomatoes, cucumber and feta in a large bowl.

2 In another bowl, whisk together the lemon juice, chilli flakes and oil to make a dressing.

3 Divide the watercress between 4 plates or shallow bowls.

4 Toast the sunflower, pumpkin and sesame seeds together in a small pan over a low heat until starting to turn golden.

5 Pour the dressing over the butter bean mixture and combine well.

6 Spoon the butter bean mixture over the watercress, then sprinkle with the toasted seeds to serve.

Butter Bean and Tomato Curry

Heat 1 tablespoon extra virgin olive oil in a pan over a medium heat, then add 1 chopped onion, 2 deseeded and chopped red peppers and 2 crushed garlic cloves and cook for 5–6 minutes. Stir in 1 teaspoon ground cumin and ½ teaspoon each of ground coriander, turmeric and chilli powder. Cook for 1–2 minutes. Stir in 4 chopped tomatoes and 2 × 400 g (13 oz) cans of butter beans, drained and rinsed. Mash a few of the butter beans, then cover the pan and simmer for 8–10 minutes. Stir in a peeled and grated 5 cm (2 inch) piece of fresh root ginger and a pinch of garam masala and cook for a further 2–3 minutes. Stir in 2 tablespoons chopped coriander. Serve with steamed basmati rice.

Roasted Butternut, Sage and Cashew Soup

Serves 4

1 kg (2 lb) butternut squash, peeled,
    deseeded and chopped into 1 cm
    (½ inch) chunks
2 tablespoons extra virgin olive oil
1 tablespoon chopped sage
2 tablespoons pumpkin seeds
1 onion, chopped
1 garlic clove, chopped
½ tablespoon mild curry powder
2 tablespoons cashew nuts
600 ml (1 pint) hot vegetable stock
8 tablespoons natural yogurt
salt and pepper

1 Place the butternut squash in a roasting tin and toss with
1 tablespoon of the oil and the sage. Place in a preheated oven, 220°C
(425°F), Gas Mark 7, for 18–20 minutes until tender and golden.

2 Meanwhile, heat a nonstick frying pan over a medium–low heat and
dry-fry the pumpkin seeds for 2–3 minutes, stirring frequently, until
golden brown and toasted. Set aside.

3 Heat the remaining oil in a saucepan, add the onion and garlic and
cook for 4–5 minutes until softened. Stir in the curry powder and cook
for a further minute, stirring.

4 Add the roasted squash, cashews and stock and bring to the boil, then
reduce the heat and simmer for 3–4 minutes. Stir in the yogurt. Using a
hand-held blender, blend the soup until smooth. Season to taste.

5 Ladle into bowls and serve sprinkled with toasted pumpkin seeds.

Butternut, Sage and Cashew Dip

Cook 300 g (10 oz) peeled, deseeded and finely diced butternut squash in
boiling water for 6–7 minutes until tender. Drain and cool for 1 minute.
Meanwhile, dry-fry 100 g (3½ oz) cashew nuts until golden. Place in a
food processor or blender with 1 tablespoon tahini and 2 garlic cloves and
blend until smooth. Add the squash, the juice of ½–1 lime, ½ tablespoon
chopped sage and a pinch of chilli powder. Season, then blend with
1–2 tablespoons extra virgin olive oil to the desired consistency.

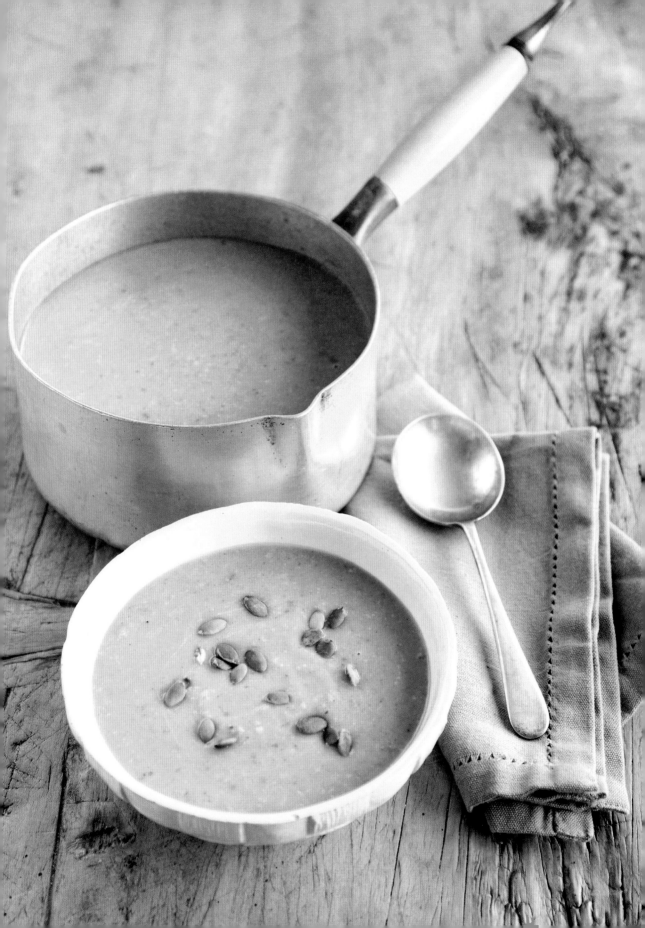

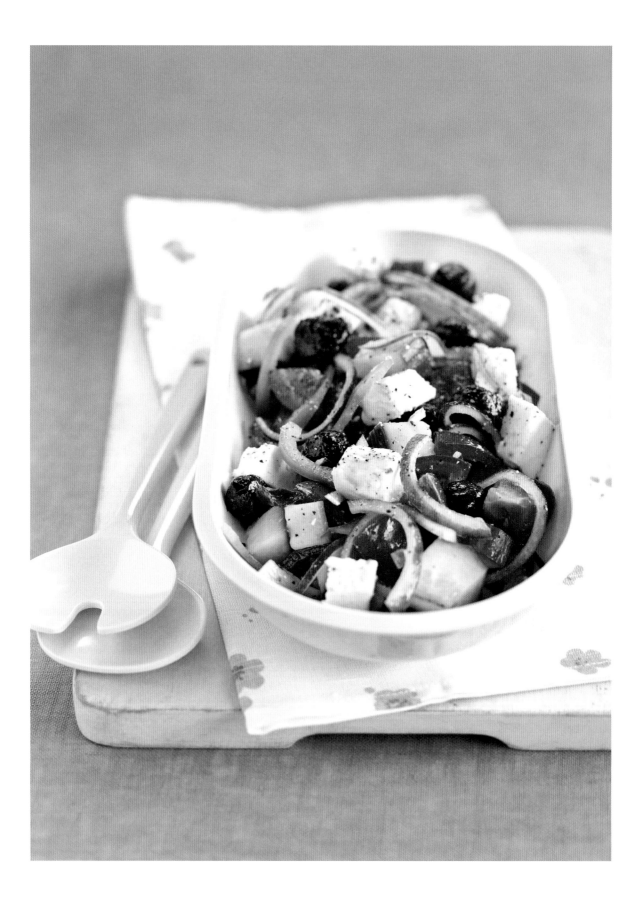

Greek Salad

Serves 2

½ cucumber, cut into 1–2 cm
    (½–¾ inch) chunks
4 plum tomatoes, cut into 1–2 cm
    (½–¾ inch) chunks
1 red pepper, cored, deseeded
    and thinly sliced
1 green pepper, cored, deseeded
    and thinly sliced
½ red onion, finely sliced
60 g (2¼ oz) pitted Kalamata olives
50 g (2 oz) feta cheese, diced

Dressing
4 tablespoons extra virgin olive oil
1 tablespoon chopped parsley
salt and pepper

Tip: When buying
Kalamata olives, look
out for those without
acidity regulators.

1 Put the cucumber and tomato chunks in a large salad bowl with
the sliced peppers, red onion and olives.

2 Make the dressing by whisking together the oil and parsley.
Season to taste with salt and pepper.

3 Pour the dressing over the salad and toss carefully. Transfer to
2 serving bowls, scatter some feta evenly over each bowl and serve.

Vietnamese-style Noodle Salad

Serves 4

200 g (7 oz) fine rice noodles
    (non-instant)
½ cucumber, deseeded and cut
    into matchsticks
1 carrot, cut into matchsticks
150 g (5 oz) bean sprouts
125 g (4 oz) mangetout, cut into
    thin strips
2 tablespoons chopped coriander
2 tablespoons chopped mint
1 red chilli, deseeded and finely sliced
2 tablespoons chopped unsalted
    peanuts, to garnish

Dressing
1 tablespoon vegetable oil
½ teaspoon caster sugar
1 tablespoon organic Thai fish sauce
2 tablespoons lime juice

1 Bring a large saucepan of water to the boil, then turn off the heat
and add the rice noodles.

2 Cover and leave to cook for 4 minutes, or according to the packet
instructions, until just tender. Drain the noodles and cool immediately
in a bowl of ice-cold water.

3 Meanwhile, make the dressing by placing the ingredients in a
screw-top jar, adding the lid and shaking until the sugar has dissolved.

4 Drain the noodles and return them to the bowl. Pour over half
of the dressing, then tip in the vegetables, herbs and chilli. Toss until
well combined.

5 Heap the noodle salad into 4 serving bowls and drizzle with the
remaining dressing. Serve scattered with the chopped peanuts.

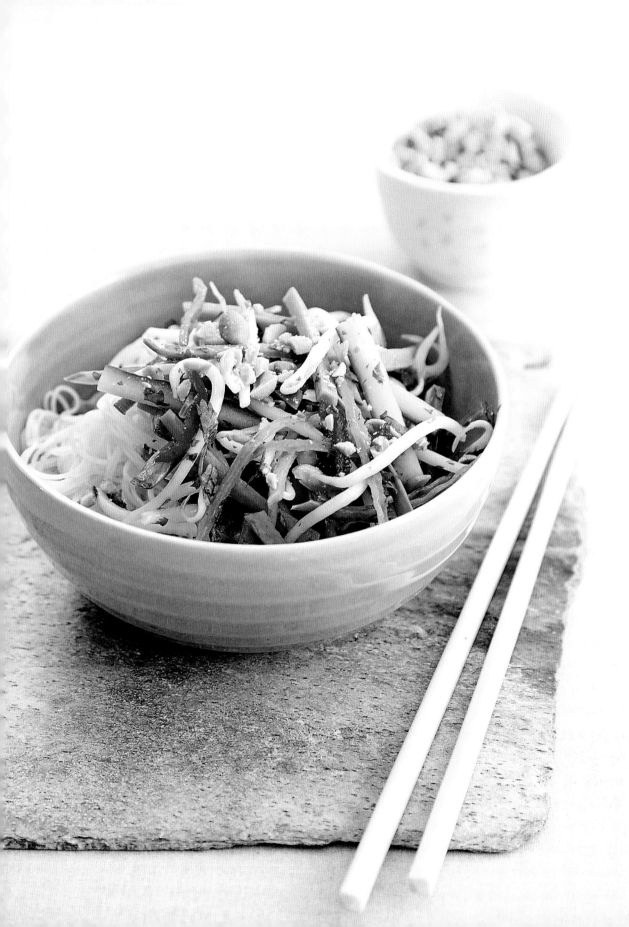

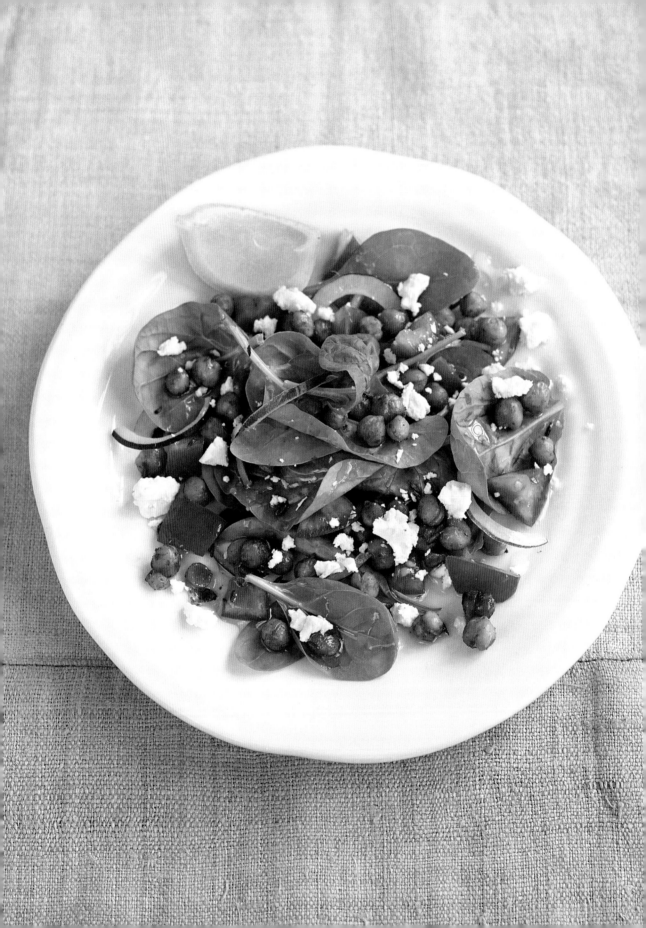

Roasted Chickpeas with Spinach

Serves 4

400 g (13 oz) can chickpeas, drained
   and rinsed
3 tablespoons extra virgin olive oil
   or vegetable oil
1 teaspoon cumin seeds
1 teaspoon paprika
½ red onion, thinly sliced
3 ripe tomatoes, roughly chopped
100 g (3½ oz) young spinach leaves
100 g (3½ oz) feta cheese (optional)
2 tablespoons lemon juice
lemon wedges, to garnish
salt and pepper

1 Mix the chickpeas in a bowl with 1 tablespoon of the oil, the cumin seeds and the paprika, and season with salt and pepper. Tip into a large nonstick roasting tin and roast in a preheated oven, 220°C (425°F), Gas Mark 7, for 12–15 minutes, until nutty and golden.

2 Meanwhile, place the onion and tomatoes in a large bowl with the spinach leaves and toss gently to combine. Heap on to 4 serving plates.

3 Remove the chickpeas from the oven and scatter over the spinach salad. Crumble the feta over the top (if using) and drizzle each plate with the lemon juice and remaining oil. Garnish with lemon wedges and serve immediately.

Aromatic Chickpea and Spinach Stew

Heat 2 tablespoons extra virgin olive oil or vegetable oil in a large, deep-sided frying pan or casserole. Chop 1 red onion, 2 large garlic cloves and a 1.5 cm (¾ inch) piece of fresh root ginger. Add to the pan and cook gently for about 10 minutes, until softened and lightly golden. Add 1 teaspoon each of cumin seeds and paprika, and cook for a further minute, then add 4 large, ripe, diced tomatoes, 400 g (13 oz) can chickpeas, drained and rinsed, 2 tablespoons lemon juice and 125 ml (4 fl oz) hot water or vegetable stock. Bring to the boil, reduce the heat and simmer gently, covered, for 12–15 minutes, until softened and thickened. Season to taste, then stir in 100 g (3½ oz) young spinach leaves, torn, and cook gently until wilted. Spoon into 4 shallow bowls and serve scattered with 2 tablespoons chopped parsley and 100 g (3½ oz) feta cheese, crumbled, if desired.

Summer Vegetable Tortiglioni with Basil Vinaigrette

Serves 4

2 tablespoons extra virgin olive oil
1 red pepper, cored, deseeded
   and sliced
1 aubergine, sliced
1 courgette, sliced
150 g (5 oz) baby plum tomatoes,
   halved
400 g (13 oz) tortiglioni
25 g (1 oz) toasted pine nuts, to serve

Basil vinaigrette
1 tablespoon white wine vinegar
½ teaspoon Dijon mustard (see tip,
   page 100)
2 tablespoons extra virgin olive oil
large handful of basil leaves,
   finely chopped
salt and pepper

1 Rub the oil over the red pepper, aubergine, courgette and tomatoes and season well. Heat a griddle pan until smoking, then add the vegetables and cook in batches until softened and lightly charred.

2 Meanwhile, cook the pasta in a large saucepan of salted boiling water according to the packet instructions until al dente. Drain the pasta, reserving a little of the cooking water.

3 To make the vinaigrette, whisk together the vinegar and mustard in a small bowl. Slowly drizzle in the oil, whisking all the time, until a smooth vinaigrette forms. Season and stir in the basil. Alternatively, make the vinaigrette in a small food processor or blender.

4 Return the pasta to the pan. Stir through a little of the vinaigrette and the griddled vegetables, adding a little cooking water to loosen if needed.

5 Spoon into serving bowls and drizzle over the remaining vinaigrette. Serve scattered with the pine nuts.

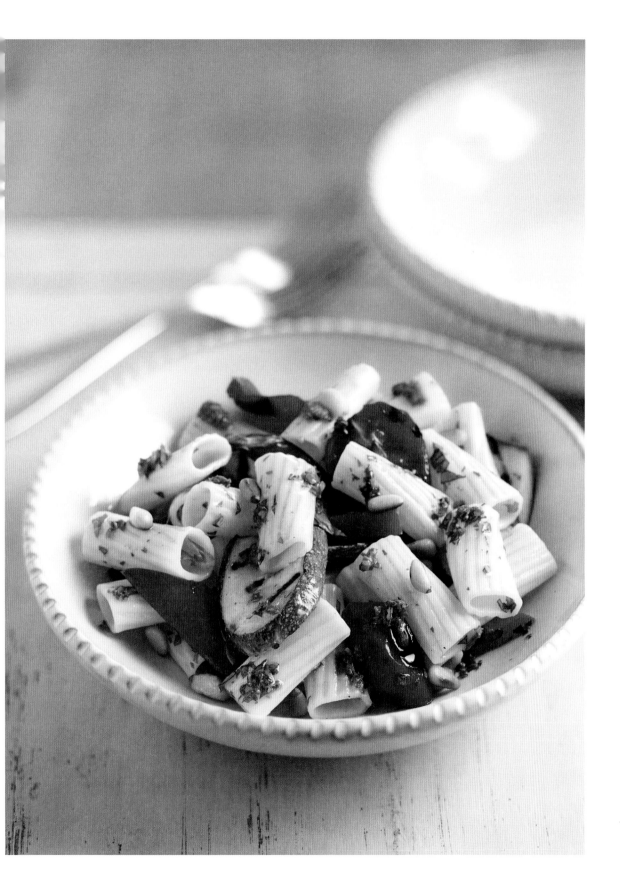

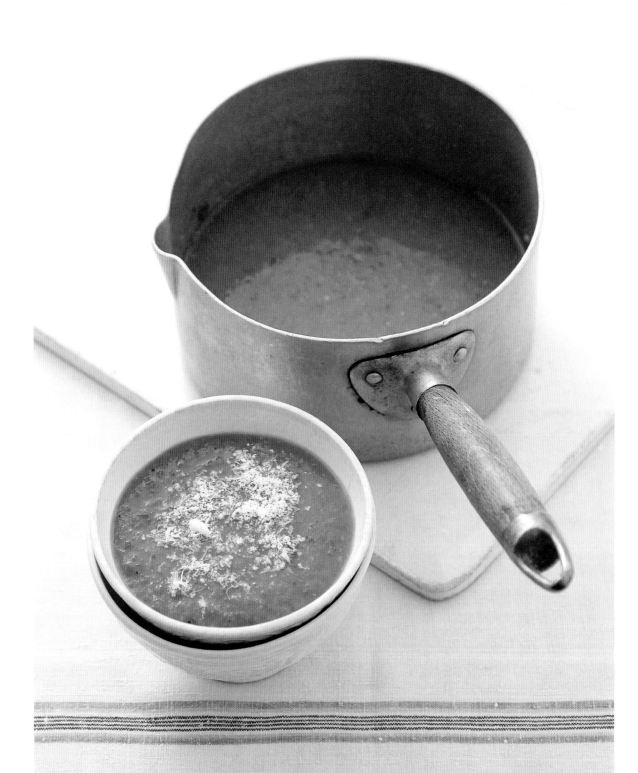

Roasted Tomato Soup

Serves 4

1 kg (2 lb) ripe tomatoes, halved
4 garlic cloves, unpeeled
2 tablespoons extra virgin olive oil
1 onion, chopped
1 carrot, chopped
1 celery stick, sliced
1 red pepper, cored, deseeded
   and chopped
700 ml (1 pint 3 fl oz) hot vegetable
   stock
salt and pepper
4 tablespoons grated Parmesan
   cheese, to serve

1 Place the tomato halves and garlic cloves in a roasting tin. Sprinkle with 1 tablespoon of the oil and some pepper and roast in a preheated oven, 200°C (400°F), Gas Mark 6, for 20 minutes.

2 After 10 minutes, heat the remaining oil in a saucepan and sauté the onion, carrot, celery and red pepper over a low heat for 10 minutes.

3 When the tomatoes are cooked, remove the garlic cloves in their skins and squeeze the garlic flesh into the pan with the vegetables.

4 Pour in the roast tomatoes and all the juices along with the stock. Using a hand-held blender, or in a food processor or blender, blend the soup until smooth. Season to taste.

5 Reheat if necessary, then serve sprinkled with the grated Parmesan.

Quick Tomato Soup

Heat 2 tablespoons extra virgin olive oil in a saucepan and sauté 1 chopped onion, 1 chopped carrot, 1 celery stick and 700 g (1½ lb) chopped tomatoes for 5 minutes. Pour in a 400 g (13 oz) can chopped tomatoes and 900 ml (1½ pints) hot vegetable stock. Simmer for 10 minutes, remove from the heat and add a small handful of basil leaves. Using a hand-held blender, or in a food processor or blender, blend the soup until smooth. Season to taste and serve with an extra drizzle of extra virgin olive oil.

Chicken, Apricot and Almond Salad

Serves 4

200 g (7 oz) celery
75 g (3 oz) almonds
3 tablespoons chopped parsley
4 tablespoons mayonnaise
3 poached or roasted chicken breasts,
    each about 150 g (5 oz)
12 fresh apricots
salt and pepper

1 Thinly slice the celery sticks diagonally, reserving the yellow inner leaves. Transfer to a large salad bowl together with half the leaves. Roughly chop the almonds and add half to the bowl with the parsley and mayonnaise. Season to taste with salt and pepper.

2 Arrange the salad on a serving plate. Shred the chicken and halve and stone the apricots. Add the chicken and apricots to the salad and stir lightly to combine.

3 Garnish with the remaining almonds and celery leaves and serve.

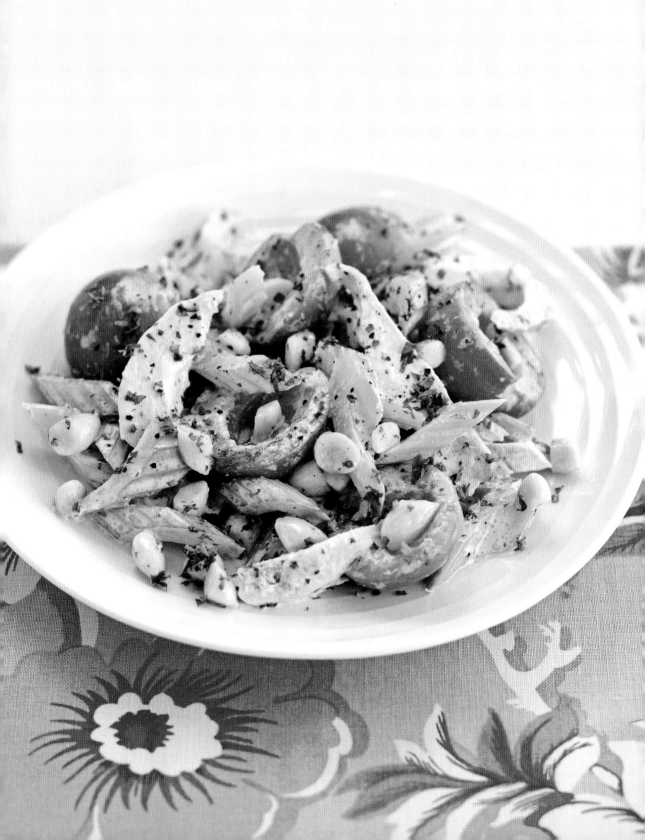

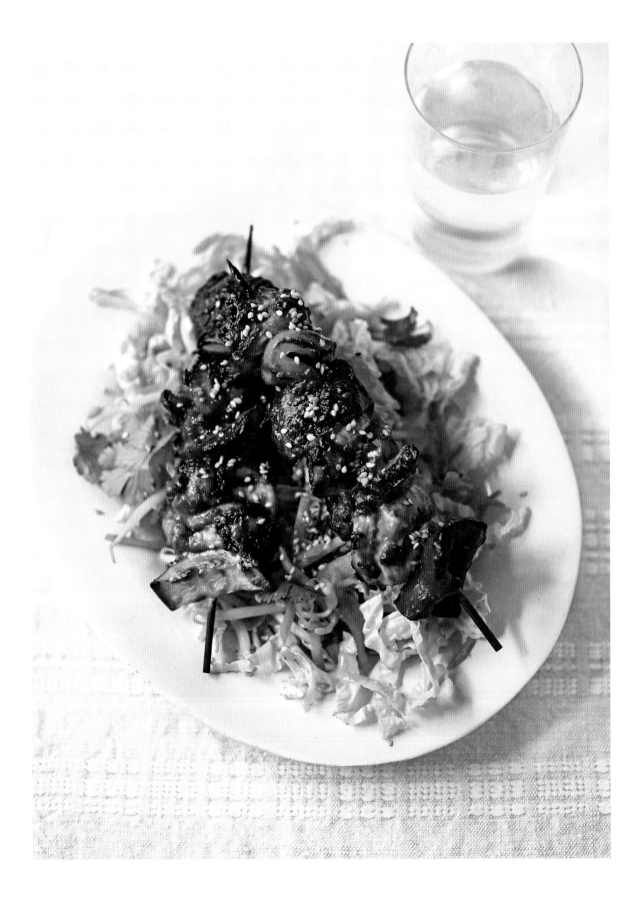

Chicken and Vegetable Satay

Serves 4

125 ml (4 fl oz) organic tamari
   soy sauce
3 tablespoons smooth additive-free
   peanut butter
2 chicken breasts, cut into strips
4 large mushrooms, halved
1 red pepper, cored, deseeded and
   cut into chunks
1 yellow pepper, cored, deseeded
   and cut into chunks
1 courgette, halved and sliced
½ Chinese lettuce, shredded
2 carrots, peeled and grated
25 g (1 oz) bean sprouts
small handful of coriander leaves
2 teaspoons sesame oil
juice of 1 lime
2 tablespoons sesame seeds,
   toasted, to serve

Tip: Seek out additive-free peanut butter (containing just ground peanuts and salt). This type of peanut butter will naturally separate, so you'll need to give it a quick stir before use.

1 In a large bowl, mix together the tamari, peanut butter and 2 tablespoons water.

2 Toss the chicken, mushrooms, peppers and courgette in the peanut mixture and thread onto 8 wooden skewers that have been soaked in water to prevent burning.

3 Place under a preheated hot grill and cook for 12–14 minutes, turning regularly, until the chicken is cooked through.

4 Meanwhile, toss together the lettuce, grated carrot, bean sprouts and coriander leaves with the sesame oil and lime juice.

5 Serve the satay with the salad, sprinkled with toasted sesame seeds.

Warm Potato and Mackerel Salad

Serves 4

400 g (13 oz) waxy new potatoes, halved
3 tablespoons extra virgin olive oil
2 teaspoons red wine vinegar
1 tablespoon additive-free wholegrain mustard
1 banana shallot, finely chopped
1 tablespoon rinsed and thinly sliced cornichons
2 teaspoons drained and rinsed organic capers
125 g (4 oz) cherry tomatoes, halved
2 tablespoons Kalamata olives, drained (see tip, page 65)
4 small mackerel fillets, boned and skin lightly scored
large handful of frisée lettuce leaves
salt and pepper

1 Cook the new potatoes in a large pan of salted boiling water for 12–15 minutes, until just tender. Drain, return to the pan and toss with 2 tablespoons of the oil. Add all the remaining ingredients, except the mackerel and frisée, then season to taste. Set aside.

2 Heat the remaining tablespoon of oil in a large nonstick frying pan and cook the mackerel fillets, skin-side down, for 3–4 minutes, until the flesh turns white. Gently turn them over and cook for a further minute, until lightly golden. Remove from the pan and cool slightly before flaking the flesh.

3 Arrange the frisée on serving plates and serve with the warm potato salad and flaked mackerel.

Quick Smoked Mackerel Pâté
Place 200 g (7 oz) peppered smoked mackerel fillets in a food processor or blender with 2 tablespoons crème fraîche, 150 g (5 oz) full-fat cream cheese and 2 teaspoons lemon juice. Blitz until almost smooth, then transfer to a bowl and stir in 2 tablespoons finely chopped parsley or chives. Scatter a few thinly sliced cornichons over the top to garnish, and serve with oatcakes (see page 159) or toast (see page 156).

Tip: Pickles such as cornichons and capers may contain added preservatives – compare labels so you can minimize your intake of these additives.

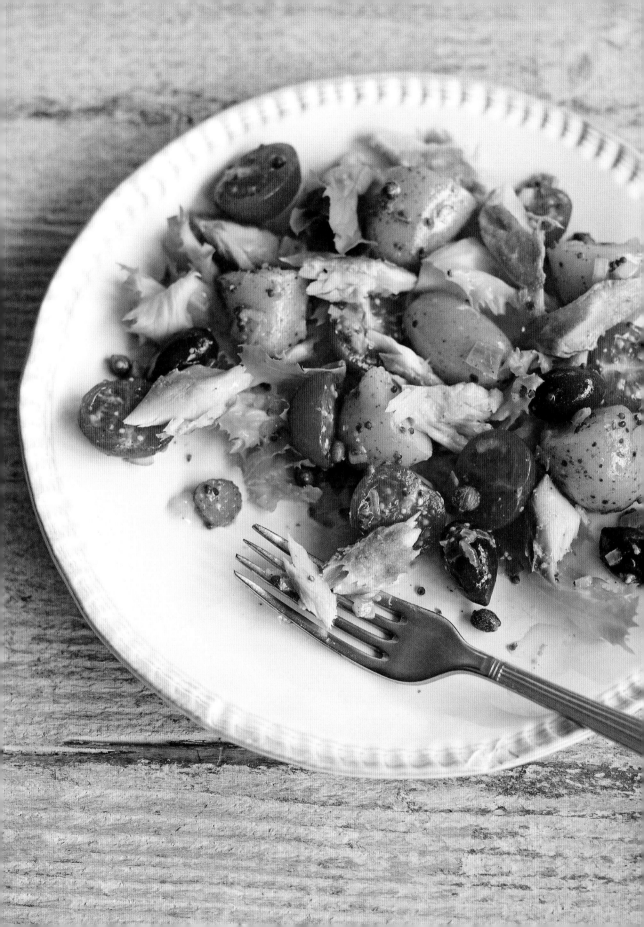

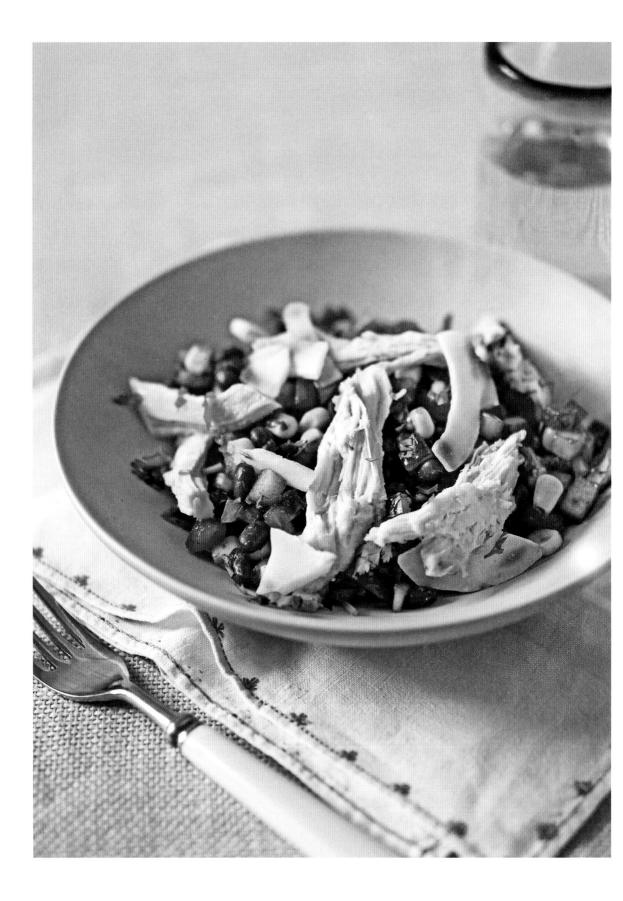

Chicken and Aduki Bean Salad

Serves 4

1 green pepper, cored, deseeded
 and chopped
1 red pepper, cored, deseeded
 and chopped
1 small red onion, finely chopped
400 g (13 oz) can aduki beans, drained
 and rinsed
200 g (7 oz) can sweetcorn, drained
small bunch of fresh coriander,
 chopped
50 g (2 oz) unsweetened organic
 coconut chips or flakes
250 g (8 oz) leftover home-cooked
 chicken breast, shredded
small handful of alfalfa shoots
 (optional)

Dressing
3 tablespoons vegetable oil
2 tablespoons organic soy sauce
2 teaspoons peeled and grated fresh
 root ginger
1 tablespoon rice vinegar

1 Mix together the green and red peppers, onion, aduki beans, sweetcorn and half the coriander in a large bowl. Whisk together the dressing ingredients in a separate bowl, then stir 3 tablespoons into the bean salad. Spoon the salad into serving dishes.

2 Place the coconut chips or flakes in a nonstick frying pan over a medium heat and dry-fry for 2–3 minutes or until lightly golden brown, stirring continuously.

3 Scatter the shredded chicken and remaining coriander over the bean salad and sprinkle with the toasted coconut and alfalfa shoots (if using). Serve with the remaining dressing.

Chicken, Avocado and Coconut Salad
Dice the flesh of 1 firm, ripe avocado, toss in 1 tablespoon of lime juice and add to the bean salad. Serve as above.

Chicken and Tarragon Pesto Penne

Serves 4

300 g (10 oz) penne
125 ml (4 fl oz) extra virgin olive oil
75 g (3 oz) Parmesan cheese, grated
handful of tarragon leaves
75 g (3 oz) pine nuts, toasted
1 garlic clove, crushed
grated rind and juice of
    1 unwaxed lemon
3 leftover home-cooked chicken
    breasts, sliced
100 g (3½ oz) watercress
12 baby tomatoes, quartered

1 Cook the penne in a large saucepan of boiling water for 8–9 minutes, or according to the packet instructions. Drain and refresh under cold running water, then toss with 2 tablespoons of the oil.

2 Meanwhile, place the grated Parmesan, tarragon, pine nuts, garlic and lemon rind in a food processor or blender and process for 1 minute. Then, while the machine is running, gradually pour in the remaining oil to form the pesto.

3 Toss the pesto with the pasta, chicken, watercress, tomatoes and lemon juice, and serve.

Chicken and Tarragon Tagliatelle

Toss 4 × 150 g (5 oz) chicken breasts in 2 tablespoons extra virgin olive oil with 2 tablespoons chopped tarragon and pepper. Cook the chicken breasts under a preheated hot grill for 5–6 minutes on each side until cooked through. Meanwhile, cook 350 g (11½ oz) tagliatelle for 9–12 minutes or according to the packet instructions. Heat 1 tablespoon extra virgin olive oil in a large frying pan over a medium heat, add 4 chopped spring onions and 12 quartered baby tomatoes and cook for 2 minutes. Slice the chicken breasts and add to the pan. Drain the pasta and toss in the pan. Serve sprinkled with 2 tablespoons toasted pine nuts.

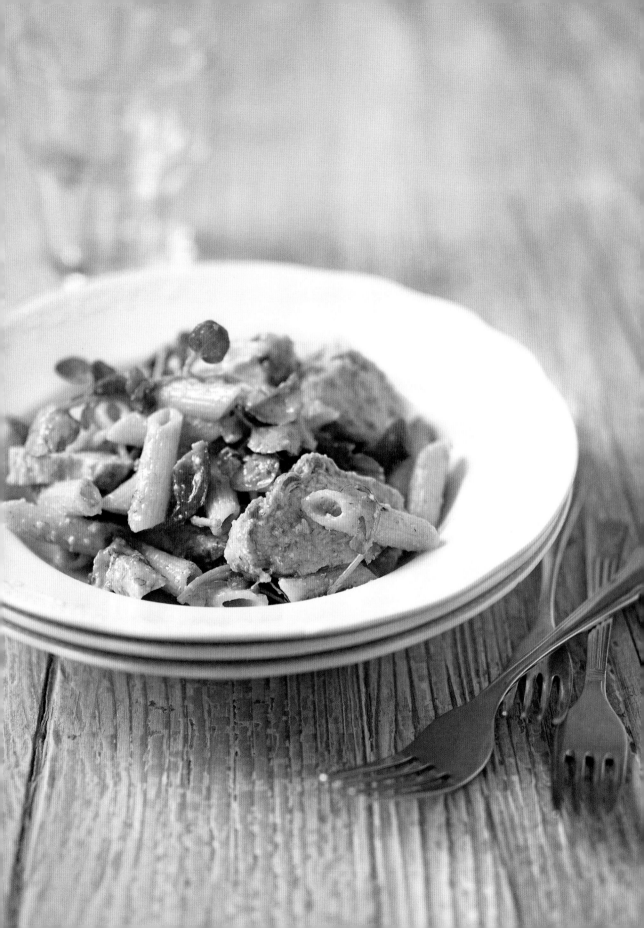

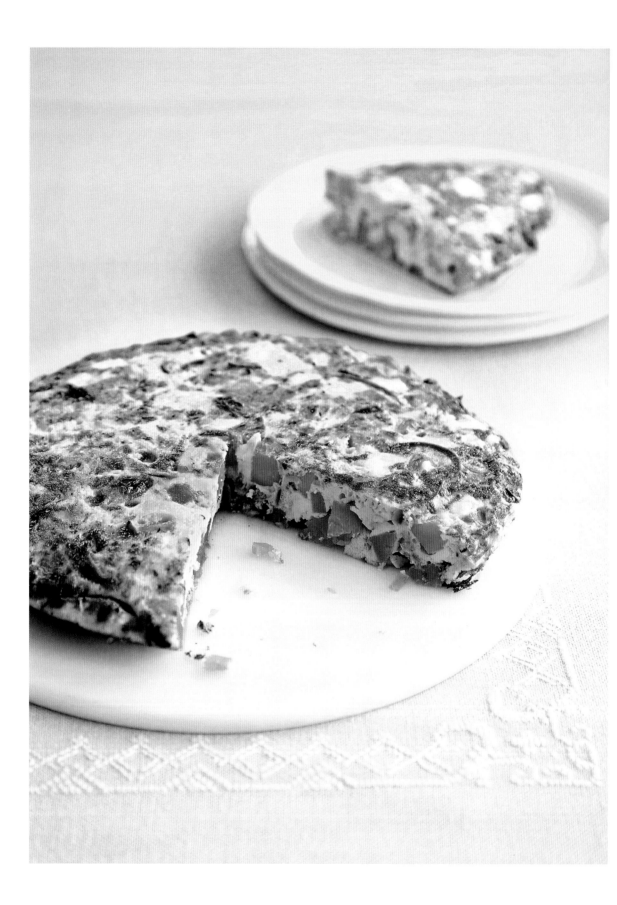

Butternut Squash and Ricotta Frittata

Serves 6

1 tablespoon extra virgin olive oil
1 red onion, thinly sliced
450 g (14½ oz) peeled and deseeded
   butternut squash, diced
8 eggs
2 tablespoons chopped sage
1 tablespoon chopped thyme
125 g (4 oz) ricotta cheese
salt and pepper

1 Heat the oil in a large, deep ovenproof frying pan over a medium–low heat, add the onion and squash, then cover loosely and cook gently, stirring frequently, for 18–20 minutes until softened and golden.

2 Beat together the eggs, herbs and ricotta lightly in a jug, then season well with salt and pepper and pour over the squash mixture.

3 Cook for 2–3 minutes until the egg is almost set, stirring occasionally to prevent the base from burning.

4 Slide the pan under a preheated medium grill, keeping the handle away from the heat, and cook for 3–4 minutes until the egg is set and the frittata is golden. Slice into 6 wedges and serve hot.

Poached Egg-topped Butternut Salad

Toss the diced butternut squash and thickly sliced red onion in the extra virgin olive oil in a roasting tin and roast in a preheated oven, 200°C (400°F), Gas Mark 6, for 20 minutes. Remove from the oven and leave to cool while you poach the eggs. Bring a saucepan of water to the boil, swirl the water with a spoon and crack in an egg, allowing the white to wrap around the yolk. Simmer for 3 minutes, then remove and keep warm. Repeat with 5 more eggs. Toss the warm roasted squash and onion with 125 g (4 oz) baby spinach leaves and divide between 6 serving plates. Top each salad with a poached egg, then spoon a little ricotta over each, sprinkle with the herbs and serve.

Dinners

Fiorentina Pizzas

Serves 4

2 tablespoons extra virgin olive oil
2 garlic cloves, sliced
1 red onion, sliced
500 g (1 lb) spinach leaves
500 g (1 lb) passata (see tip, page 49)
4–8 eggs
2 tablespoons pine nuts
200 g (7 oz) mozzarella cheese,
    freshly grated
pepper

Pizza dough
1 kg (2 lb) strong white bread flour
2 × 7 g (¼ oz) sachets fast-action
    dried yeast (see page 18)
2 tablespoons extra virgin olive oil
600 ml (1 pint) warm water, plus
    1–2 tablespoons
salt

1 First make the pizza dough. Mix together the strong bread flour, yeast and a pinch of salt. Stir in 1–2 tablespoons warm water. Mix together with your hand, gradually adding about 600 ml (1 pint) warm water, until you have a soft, but not sticky dough.

2 Turn the dough out onto a lightly floured work surface and knead for 5–8 minutes, until the dough is smooth and elastic. Divide into 4 pieces and roll into 30 cm (12 inch) circles, then place on 2 baking trays.

3 Heat the oil in a large frying pan and sauté the garlic and onion for 2–3 minutes, then add the spinach and stir until it has completely wilted. Set aside.

4 Spread the passata over the pizza bases, followed by the spinach and make a small hollow in each pizza topping. Break 1–2 eggs into the hollows. Sprinkle each pizza with pine nuts, mozzarella and pepper.

5 Bake in a preheated oven, 220°C (425°F), Gas Mark 7, for 6–7 minutes, until the eggs are cooked.

Tip: Shop-bought grated mozzarella tends to have added starch to keeps the flakes separate, so it's better to opt for a ball of fresh mozzarella. To make it easier to grate, pop the mozzarella in the freezer for 10–15 minutes before grating.

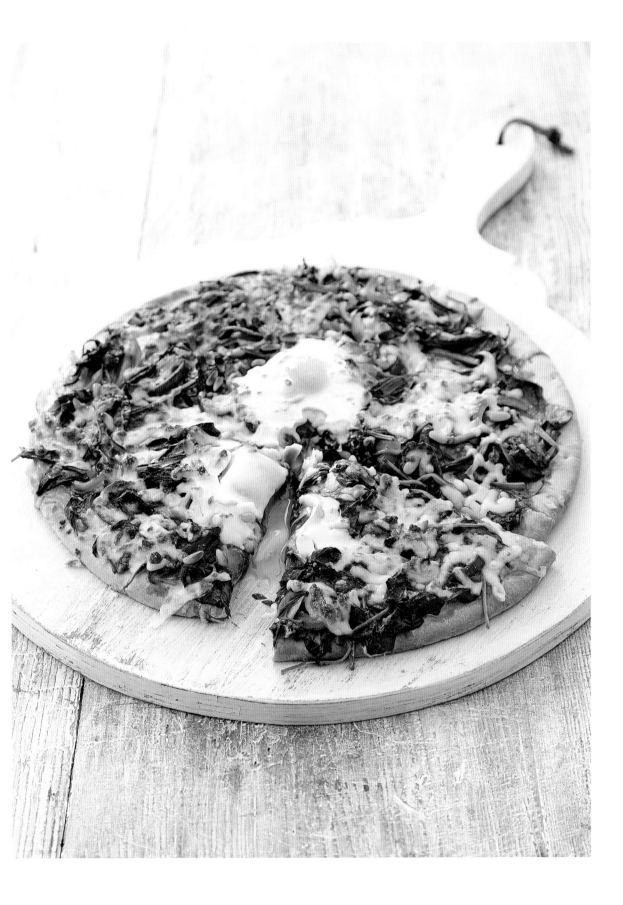

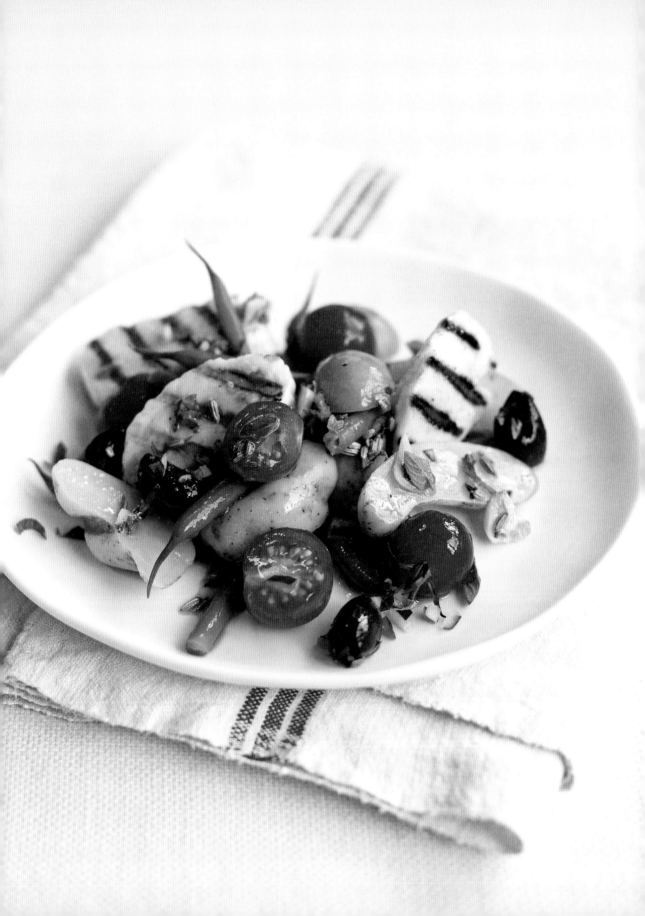

Chargrilled Halloumi with Roasted Olives and Salad

Serves 4

3 garlic cloves
6 tablespoons extra virgin olive oil
pinch of dried chilli flakes
finely grated rind and juice of
   ½ unwaxed orange
1 teaspoon fennel seeds
100 g (3½ oz) pitted black olives
300 g (10 oz) salad potatoes, halved
150 g (5 oz) green beans
250 g (8 oz) halloumi cheese,
   thickly sliced
1 tablespoon red wine vinegar
125 g (4 oz) cherry tomatoes, halved
½ red onion, chopped
handful of oregano leaves, chopped
salt and pepper

1 Slice 2 of the garlic cloves and mix together with 2 tablespoons of the oil, the chilli, orange rind and juice, fennel seeds and olives. Place on a small baking tray and cook in a preheated oven, 200°C (400°F), Gas Mark 6, for 15 minutes.

2 Meanwhile, cook the potatoes in a large saucepan of boiling water for 10 minutes, then add the beans and cook for 3–5 minutes more until soft. Drain and cool under cold running water. Heat a griddle pan until smoking. Pat the halloumi dry and griddle for 2–3 minutes on each side until golden and lightly charred.

3 Crush the remaining garlic and whisk together with the vinegar and the remaining oil. Toss the dressing together with the potatoes and beans, tomatoes and onion. Arrange on a plate with the halloumi slices, drizzle over the warm olives and marinade, then scatter over the oregano to serve.

Pea and Mint Risotto

Serves 4

1 tablespoon extra virgin olive oil
2 shallots, finely diced
400 g (13 oz) Arborio rice
100 ml (3½ fl oz) white wine
about 900 ml (1½ pints) hot
   vegetable stock
100 g (3½ oz) fresh or frozen
   peas, defrosted
a small handful of mint leaves,
   chopped
40 g (1¾ oz) butter
40 g (1¾ oz) Parmesan cheese, grated
salt and pepper

1 Heat the oil in a large saucepan and sauté the shallots for 2–3 minutes, until softened but not coloured.

2 Stir in the rice and continue to stir, until the edges of the grains look translucent. Pour in the wine and cook for 1–2 minutes, until it is absorbed.

3 Add a ladle of the hot vegetable stock and stir continuously, until it has all been absorbed.

4 Repeat with the remaining hot stock, adding a ladle at a time, until the rice is al dente.

5 Stir in the peas, mint, butter and half the grated Parmesan, season with salt and pepper and cook for a further 2–3 minutes.

6 Serve sprinkled with the remaining Parmesan.

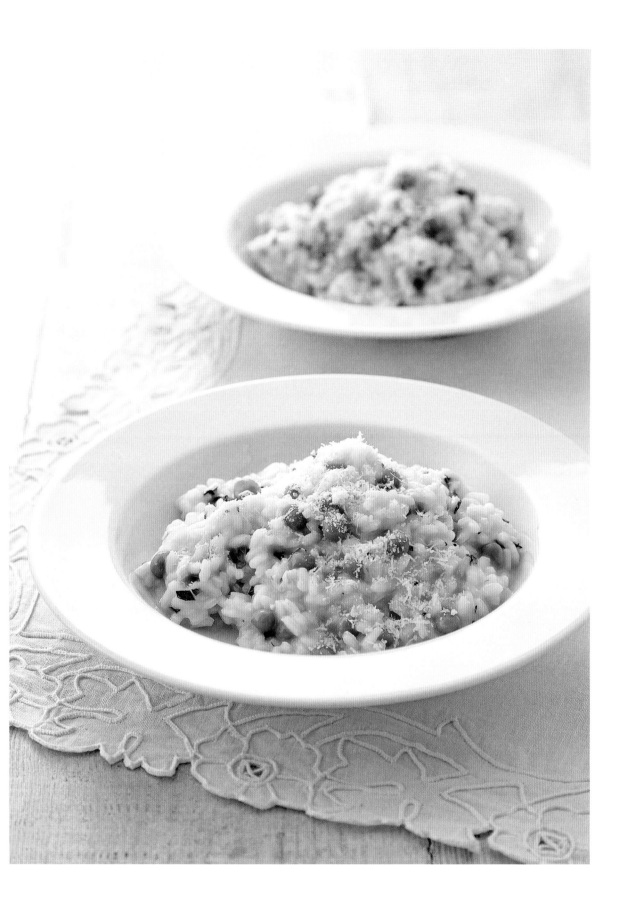

Frying Pan Macaroni Cheese

Serves 4

325 g (11 oz) macaroni
50 g (2 oz) butter
50 g (2 oz) plain flour
600 ml (1 pint) milk
100 g (3½ oz) Cheddar cheese, grated
25 g (1 oz) Panko breadcrumbs
25 g (1 oz) Parmesan cheese, grated
salt and pepper

1 Cook the pasta in a large saucepan of salted boiling water according to the packet instructions until al dente.

2 Meanwhile, melt the butter in a large, ovenproof frying pan and stir in the flour to make a smooth paste. Cook until golden, then gradually whisk in the milk. Bring to the boil over a medium heat, then simmer for about 3 minutes until slightly thickened. Remove from the heat, stir in the Cheddar and season.

3 Drain the pasta, then tip into the frying pan. Stir into the cheese sauce until well combined. Scatter over the breadcrumbs and Parmesan.

4 Place in a preheated oven, 190°C (375°F), Gas Mark 5, for 15 minutes or until golden brown and bubbling.

Tip: Panko breadcrumbs are made with just wheat flour, yeast and salt, making a delish crunchy (UPF-free) topping.

Pasta in a Cheesy Sauce

Cook 400 g (13 oz) chifferi pasta according to the packet instructions until al dente. Meanwhile, place 1 garlic clove and 100 ml (3½ fl oz) double cream in a saucepan and cook for 5 minutes. Remove and discard the garlic and stir in 50 g (2 oz) grated Parmesan. Drain the pasta and return to the pan. Stir through the sauce and serve immediately.

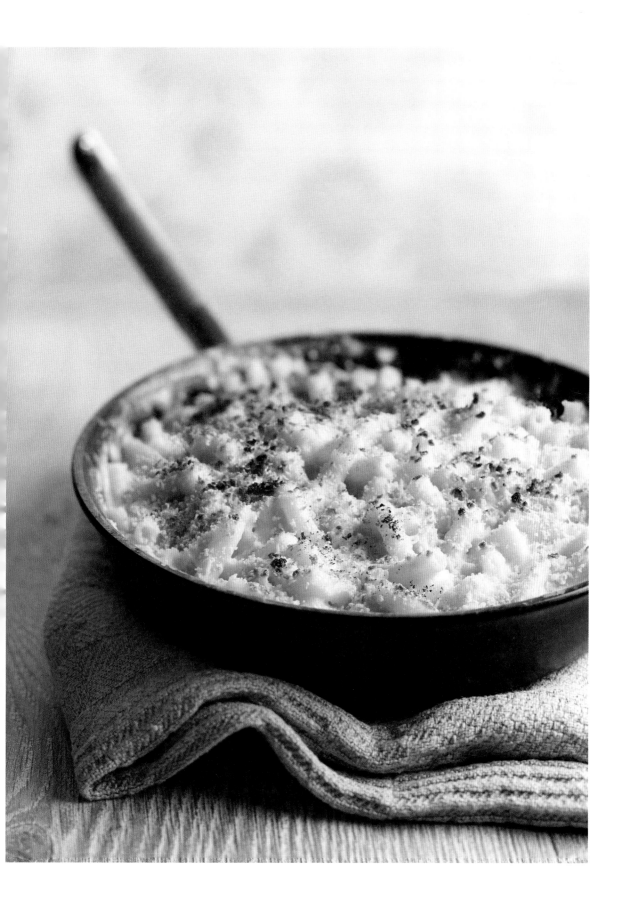

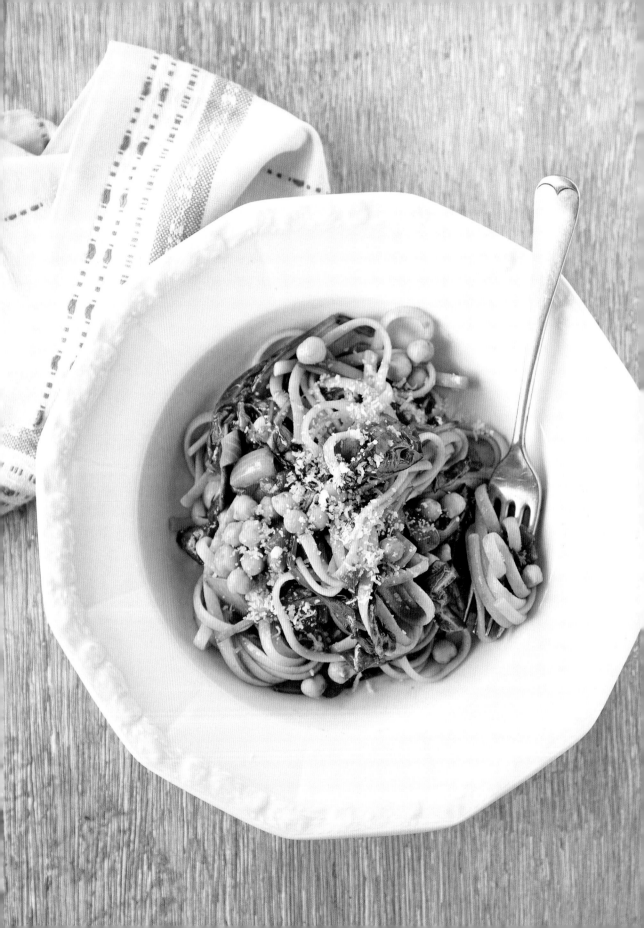

Linguine with Chickpea and Tomato Sauce

Serves 4

2 tablespoons extra virgin olive oil
1 onion, chopped
2 garlic cloves, crushed
1 celery stick, sliced
400 g (13 oz) can chopped tomatoes
175 g (6 oz) baby spinach leaves
400 g (13 oz) can chickpeas, drained
    and rinsed
350 g (11½ oz) linguine
10 basil leaves, torn
50 g (2 oz) Parmesan cheese, grated,
    to serve

1 Heat the oil in a large saucepan, add the onion, garlic and celery and cook for 3–4 minutes until softened. Add the tomatoes and bring to the boil, then reduce the heat and simmer for 10 minutes. Stir in the spinach and chickpeas and cook until the spinach is wilted.

2 Meanwhile, cook the pasta in a saucepan of boiling water for 6–8 minutes, or according to the packet instructions, until al dente. Drain, then add to the tomato sauce with the basil and toss together.

3 Serve sprinkled with the grated Parmesan.

Chickpea, Tomato and Pasta Salad
Cook 300 g (10 oz) farfalle in a saucepan of boiling water for 7–8 minutes, or according to the packet instructions, until al dente. Drain, then refresh under cold running water and drain again. Place in a serving bowl and toss together with a drained and rinsed 400 g (13 oz) can chickpeas, 1 diced red onion, 4 chopped tomatoes, 6 torn basil leaves, 50 g (2 oz) rocket leaves, 2 tablespoons Parmesan shavings, 2 tablespoons extra virgin olive oil and 1 tablespoon balsamic vinegar. Season to taste and serve.

Moroccan-inspired Vegetable Stew

Serves 4

1 tablespoon extra virgin olive oil
1 onion, chopped
2 garlic cloves, chopped
375 g (12 oz) sweet potatoes,
   peeled and chopped
175 g (6 oz) parsnips, chopped
275 g (9 oz) swede, chopped
2 large carrots, chopped
250 g (8 oz) Brussels sprouts
½ teaspoon ground cumin
1 teaspoon ground coriander
½ teaspoon turmeric
¼ teaspoon cayenne pepper
½ teaspoon ground cinnamon
400 g (13 oz) can chopped tomatoes
400 ml (14 fl oz) vegetable stock
cooked couscous, to serve

1 Heat the oil in a large, heavy-based saucepan, add the onion
and garlic and fry for 2–3 minutes. Add the remaining vegetables,
reduce the heat to low and cook, stirring occasionally, for 2–3 minutes
without browning.

2 Add the spices and mix well to coat all the vegetables, then pour
in the tomatoes and vegetable stock. Bring to the boil, then reduce
the heat and simmer, breaking up the tomatoes with a wooden
spoon, for 20–22 minutes or until the vegetables are tender.

3 Serve with couscous to soak up the juices.

Moroccan-inspired Vegetable Soup

Heat 1 tablespoon extra virgin olive oil in a saucepan, add 1 sliced red
onion and 2 diced garlic cloves and cook for 1 minute. Stir in ½ teaspoon
each of turmeric and ground cumin, ¼ teaspoon cayenne pepper and
a pinch of ground cinnamon. Add 1 peeled, diced sweet potato, 2 cored,
deseeded and sliced red peppers and ½ savoy cabbage, shredded. Pour
in 1.2 litres (2 pints) vegetable stock and bring to the boil. Reduce the
heat and simmer for 8 minutes. Blitz the soup briefly with a hand-held
blender, then serve sprinkled with toasted flaked almonds.

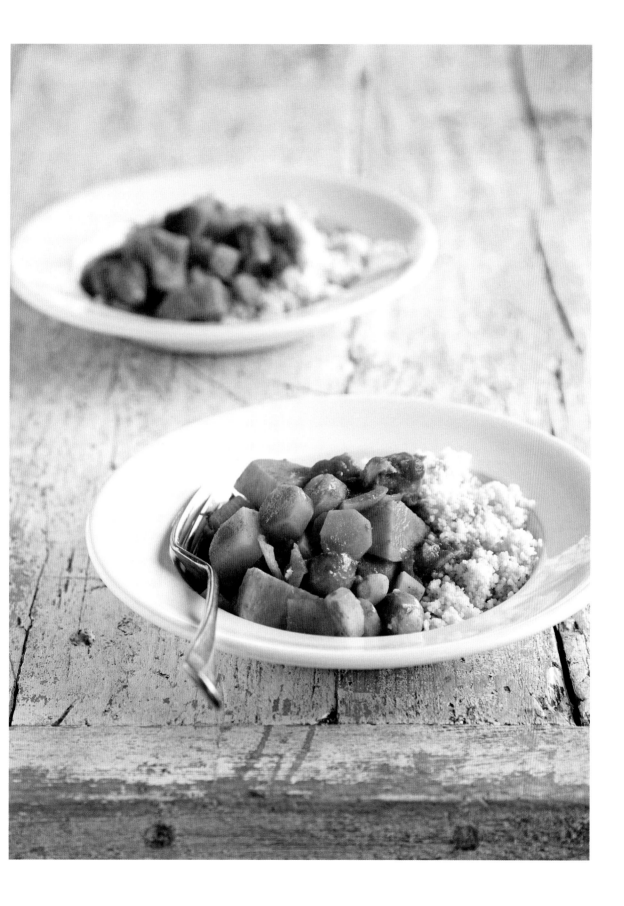

Cod Fillets with Tomatoes and Salsa Verde

Serves 4

4 thick cod fillets
4 plum tomatoes, halved
1 tablespoon extra virgin olive oil
salt and pepper

Salsa verde
2 canned anchovy fillets
1 garlic clove, peeled
1 teaspoon organic capers, drained
1 tablespoon Dijon mustard
1 tablespoon white wine vinegar
100 ml (3½ fl oz) extra virgin olive oil
large handful of parsley,
    finely chopped
large handful of basil, finely chopped

1   Season the cod and put it in a lightly greased ovenproof dish along with the tomatoes. Drizzle over the oil and cook in a preheated oven, 200°C (400°F), Gas Mark 6, for 15 minutes until the fish is opaque and just cooked through.

2   Chop the anchovies, garlic and capers very finely to form a rough paste. Mix together with the mustard and vinegar, then stir in the oil, followed by the herbs.

3   Drizzle the sauce over the fish fillets and tomatoes to serve.

Tip: Some Dijon mustards contain additives so make sure you check the label before you buy – organic versions tend to be additive-free.

Salsa Verde Cod Skewers
Cube 400 g (13 oz) thick, skinless, boneless cod fillets and toss together with 3 tablespoons extra virgin olive oil, the finely grated rind of 1 unwaxed lemon, 1 crushed garlic clove and a large handful each of chopped parsley and basil. Season well and thread on to skewers. Cook on a hot griddle for 3 minutes on each side until just cooked through. Squeeze over a little lemon juice and serve.

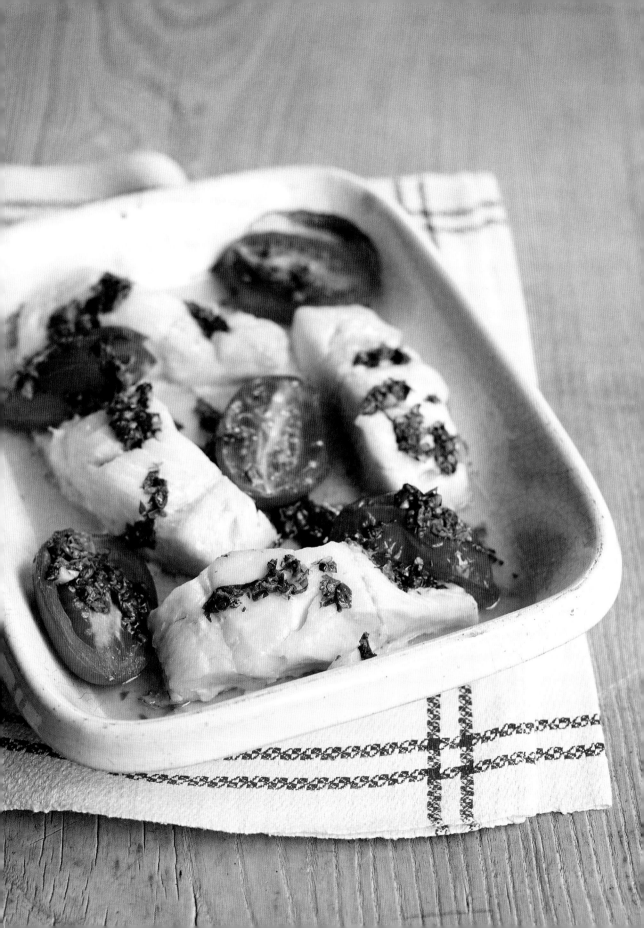

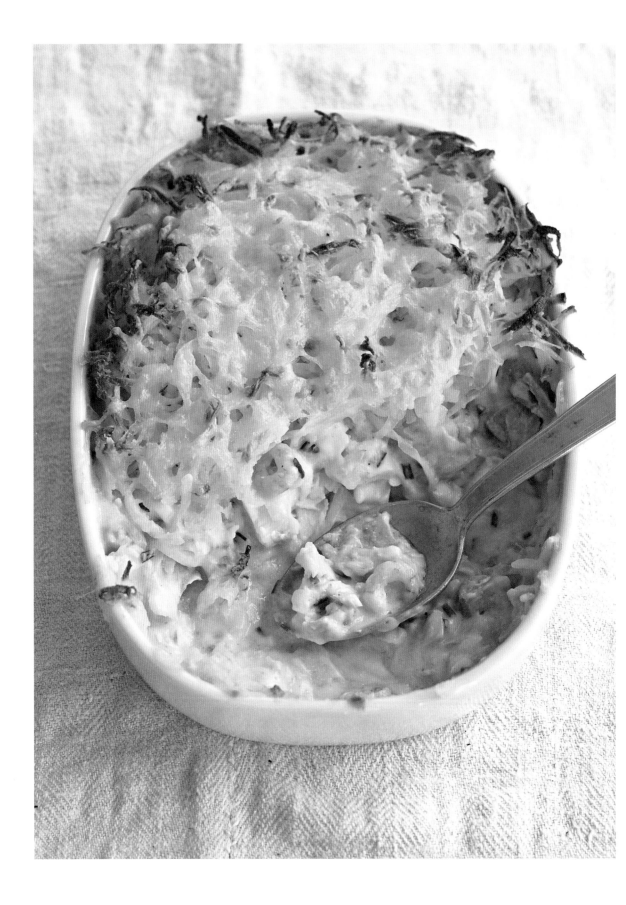

Easy Fish Pie with Crunchy Potato Topping

Serves 4

750 g (1½ lb) medium potatoes, unpeeled

250 g (8 oz) white fish fillet, such as coley, pollack or haddock, cut into bite- sized pieces

250 g (8 oz) salmon fillet, cut into bite-sized pieces

400 ml (14 fl oz) hot milk

50 g (2 oz) butter

50 g (2 oz) flour

100 g (3½ oz) Cheddar cheese, grated

2 teaspoons lemon juice

2 tablespoons chopped chives

100 g (3½ oz) small cooked peeled prawns (optional)

salt and pepper

1 Cook the potatoes in a large saucepan of lightly salted water for 6–7 minutes. Drain and set aside to cool slightly.

2 Meanwhile, place the fish in a deep-sided frying pan. Pour over the hot milk and bring to the boil. Reduce the heat and simmer gently for 3–4 minutes, until the fish is just cooked. Strain the milk into a jug and retain, and transfer the fish to an ovenproof dish.

3 Place the butter and flour in a saucepan and warm gently to melt the butter. Stir over the heat to cook the flour for 2 minutes, then add the milk a little at a time, stirring well to incorporate. Stir over the heat for 2–3 minutes, until thickened, then remove from the heat and stir in half the Cheddar, the lemon juice and chives, and season to taste. Pour the sauce over the fish, add the prawns (if using) and stir gently to coat.

4 Wearing rubber gloves to protect your hands from the heat, grate the potatoes coarsely and scatter over the fish. Sprinkle with the remaining Cheddar and cook in a preheated oven, 180°C (350°F), Gas Mark 4, for 15–20 minutes, until the topping is golden and crispy.

Keralan-style Fish Curry

Serves 4

1 red chilli, deseeded and chopped
1 teaspoon vegetable oil
1 teaspoon ground coriander
½ teaspoon ground cumin
½ teaspoon turmeric
4 garlic cloves
2.5 cm (1 inch) piece of fresh root
    ginger, peeled and chopped
1 tablespoon coconut oil
¼ teaspoon fenugreek seeds
2 onions, finely sliced
125 ml (4 fl oz) organic coconut milk
300 ml (½ pint) water
400 g (13 oz) fresh mackerel fillets,
    skinned and cut into 5-cm
    (2-inch) pieces
salt and pepper

1 Place the chilli, vegetable oil, coriander, cumin, turmeric, garlic and ginger in a mini food processor or small blender and blend to a paste.

2 Heat the coconut oil in a wok or large pan, add the paste and fenugreek seeds and fry for 2–3 minutes. Add the onions, coconut milk and measured water, season and bring to the boil, then cook for about 5 minutes until reduced.

3 Add the mackerel and simmer gently for 5–8 minutes or until cooked through.

Indian-style Spiced Fishcakes
Cook 1 kg (2 lb) peeled and chopped potatoes in a saucepan of boiling water for 15–17 minutes until tender. Meanwhile, dry-fry 1 teaspoon cumin seeds in a nonstick frying pan for 2–3 minutes, stirring, until toasted. Drain the potatoes, then mash in the pan with the cumin seeds, 2 finely chopped spring onions, 1 deseeded and diced red chilli, 3 tablespoons chopped coriander and salt and pepper. Beat in 1 beaten egg, then carefully stir in 200 g (7 oz) flaked hot-smoked salmon fillets. Using wet hands, shape into 8 fishcakes, then coat in 4 tablespoons plain flour. Heat 25 g (1 oz) butter and 1 tablespooon vegetable oil in a frying pan, add the fishcakes and fry for about 2 minutes on each side until golden. Serve with yogurt raita and a rocket salad.

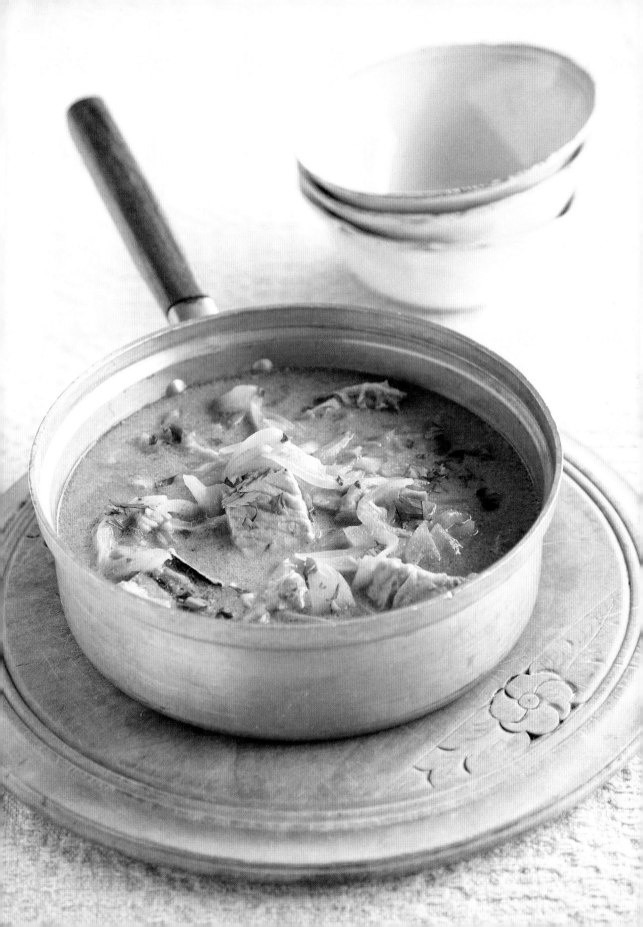

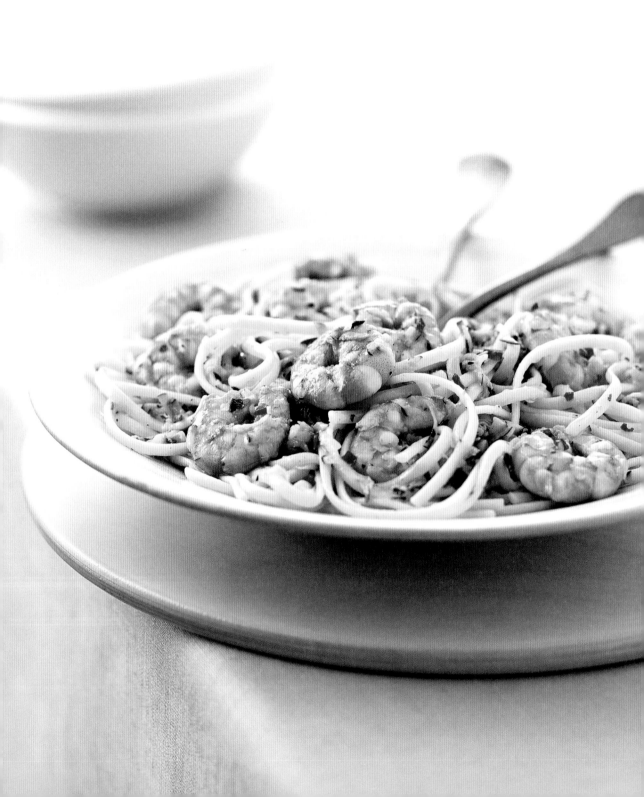

King Prawn and Courgette Linguine

Serves 4

400 g (13 oz) dried linguine
3 tablespoons extra virgin olive oil
200 g (7 oz) raw peeled king prawns
2 garlic cloves, crushed
finely grated rind of 1 unwaxed lemon
1 fresh red chilli, deseeded and
 finely chopped
400 g (13 oz) courgettes, coarsely
 grated
50 g (2 oz) unsalted butter,
 cut into cubes
salt

1 Cook the pasta in a large saucepan of salted boiling water according to the packet instructions until al dente. Drain.

2 Meanwhile, heat the oil in a large frying pan over a high heat until the surface of the oil seems to shimmer slightly. Add the prawns, garlic, lemon rind and chilli, season with salt and cook, stirring, for 2 minutes until the prawns turn pink. Add the courgettes and butter, season with a little more salt and stir well. Cook, stirring, for 30 seconds.

3 Toss in the pasta and stir until the butter has melted and all the ingredients are well combined. Serve immediately.

Chicken and Spinach Stew

Serves 4

625 g (1¼ lb) skinless, boneless
   chicken thigh, thinly sliced
2 teaspoons ground cumin
1 teaspoon ground ginger
2 tablespoons extra virgin olive oil
1 tablespoon tomato purée
2 × 400 g (13 oz) cans cherry tomatoes
50 g (2 oz) raisins
400 g (13 oz) can brown or green
   lentils, drained and rinsed
1 teaspoon grated unwaxed lemon rind
150 g (5 oz) baby spinach
salt and pepper
freshly chopped parsley, to garnish
   (optional)
steamed couscous or rice, to serve
   (optional)

1 Mix the chicken with the ground spices until well coated. Heat the oil in a large saucepan or flameproof casserole dish, then add the chicken and cook for 2–3 minutes, until lightly browned.

2 Stir in the tomato purée, tomatoes, raisins, lentils and lemon rind, season and simmer gently for about 12 minutes, until thickened slightly and the chicken is cooked through.

3 Add the spinach and stir until wilted. Ladle the stew into bowls, then scatter with parsley, if using, and serve with steamed couscous or rice, if desired.

Quick Spinach and Watercress Soup
Melt 25 g (1 oz) butter in a large saucepan and fry 1 chopped garlic clove and 2 chopped spring onions over a medium heat for 2–3 minutes. Add 175 g (6 oz) cooked, peeled new potatoes and 1 litre (1¾ pints) hot vegetable stock. Bring to a simmer, then add 150 g (5 oz) watercress and 200 g (7 oz) chopped spinach leaves. Heat for 1–2 minutes, then blend until smooth. Season, then add a pinch of ground nutmeg. Ladle into bowls and top each with crème fraîche and a dusting of grated nutmeg.

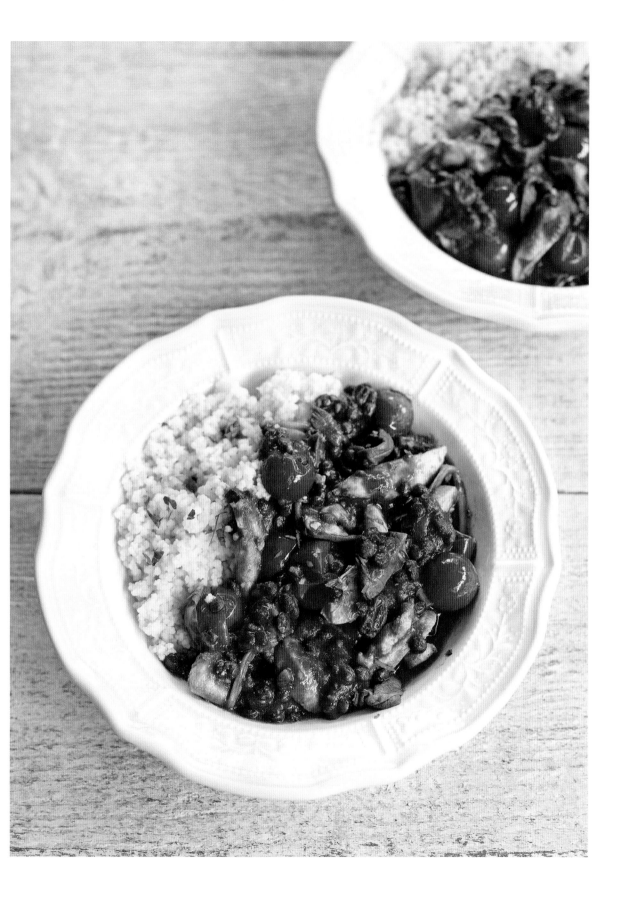

Yellow Chicken Drumstick Curry

Serves 4

2 fresh red chillies, roughly chopped,
    plus extra to garnish
2 shallots, roughly chopped
3 garlic cloves, chopped
4 tablespoons chopped lemon grass
    (outer leaves removed)
1 tablespoon peeled and finely
    chopped galangal
2 teaspoons ground turmeric
1 teaspoon cayenne pepper
1 teaspoon ground coriander
1 teaspoon ground cumin
¼ teaspoon ground cinnamon
3 tablespoons organic Thai fish sauce
1 tablespoon palm sugar or
    brown sugar
4 kaffir lime leaves, shredded
400 ml (14 fl oz) can organic
    coconut milk
juice of ½ lime
8 large chicken drumsticks, skinned
200 g (7 oz) baby new potatoes, peeled
10–12 Thai basil leaves, to garnish

1 Place the chillies, shallots, garlic, lemon grass, galangal, turmeric, cayenne pepper, coriander, cumin, cinnamon, fish sauce, sugar, lime leaves, coconut milk and lime juice in a food processor or blender, and blend until fairly smooth.

2 Arrange the chicken drumsticks in a single layer in an ovenproof casserole. Scatter over the potatoes. Pour over the spice paste to coat the chicken and potatoes evenly. Cover and cook in a preheated oven, 180°C (350°F), Gas Mark 4, for 40–45 minutes until the chicken is cooked through and the potatoes are tender. Serve hot, garnished with the basil and chopped red chilli.

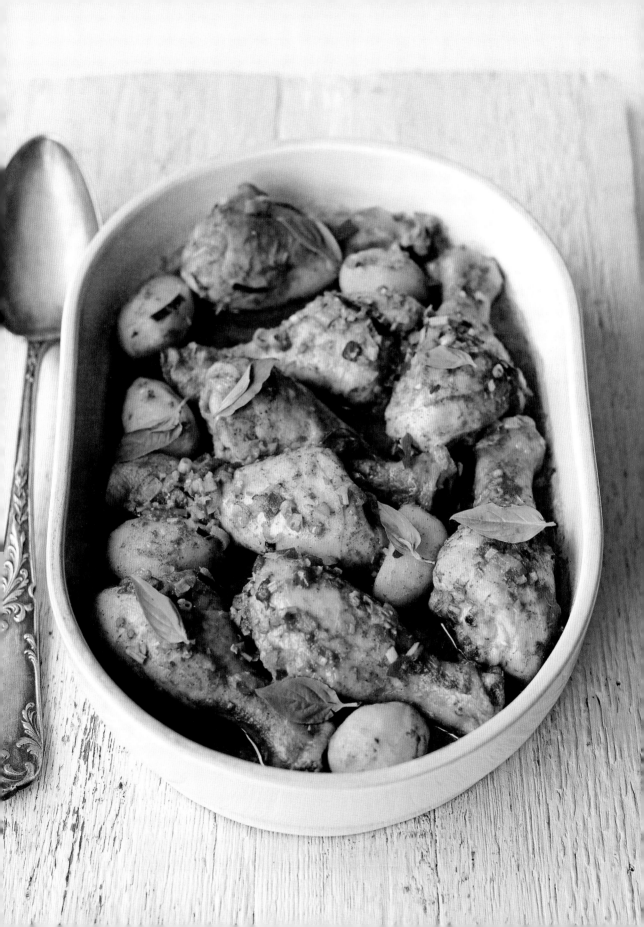

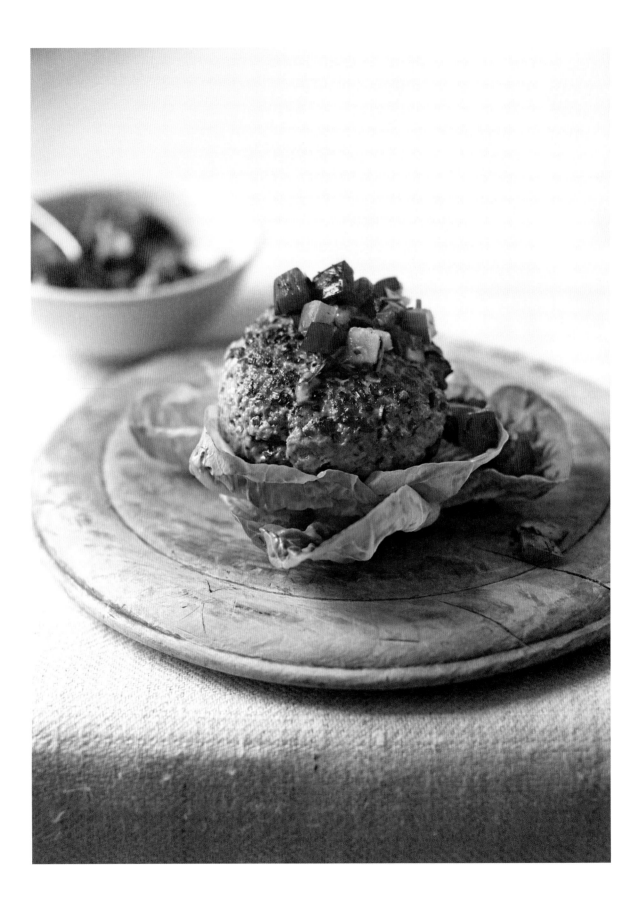

Spicy Turkey Burgers with Red Pepper Salsa

Serves 4

400 g (13 oz) minced turkey
2 cm (¾ inch) piece of fresh root
  ginger, peeled and grated
4 spring onions, finely chopped
1 red chilli, deseeded and
  finely chopped
1 egg yolk
2 tablespoons chopped
  coriander leaves
1 tablespoon vegetable oil
Little Gem lettuce leaves, to serve

Red pepper salsa
1 red pepper, cored, deseeded
  and diced
100 g (3½ oz) tomatoes, diced
1 small red onion, finely diced
½ tablespoon chopped parsley
½ tablespoon chopped
  coriander leaves
1 tablespoon red wine vinegar
½ tablespoon extra virgin olive oil

1 Mix together the minced turkey, ginger, spring onions, chilli, egg yolk and coriander.

2 Using wet hands, shape the mixture into 4 burgers.

3 Heat the vegetable oil in a frying pan and cook the burgers for 5–6 minutes on either side, until golden and cooked through.

4 Meanwhile, for the salsa, mix together the pepper, tomatoes, onion, parsley, coriander, vinegar and extra virgin olive oil.

5 Serve the burgers on a bed of lettuce leaves, topped with the salsa.

Leftover Turkey Salad

Mix together 3 finely sliced shallots with ¼ teaspoon salt and leave to stand for 10 minutes. Whisk together the juice of 1 lime, 2 tablespoons organic Thai fish sauce, 1 tablespoon rice vinegar, 1 tablespoon caster sugar, 2 crushed garlic cloves and 1 finely diced red chilli. In a large bowl, toss together 350 g (11½ oz) cooked turkey, cut into strips, 400 g (13 oz) finely shredded Chinese cabbage, 1 large peeled and grated carrot, 100 g (3½ oz) bean sprouts and a small handful each of mint and basil. Toss in the shallots and dressing and leave to stand for 5 minutes, then serve sprinkled with 50 g (2 oz) chopped roasted peanuts.

Thai Green Chicken Curry

Serves 4

400 ml (14 fl oz) can organic coconut milk

100 g (3½ oz) chopped coriander

1 tablespoon vegetable oil

3 tablespoons Thai green curry paste (see below)

2 green chillies, deseeded and finely chopped

800 g (1¾ lb) boneless, skinless chicken thighs, cut into bite-sized pieces

200 ml (7 fl oz) hot chicken stock

6 lime leaves

2 tablespoons organic Thai fish sauce

1 tablespoon grated palm sugar or caster sugar

200 g (7 oz) Thai baby aubergines, halved if large, or cut into 1.5 cm (¾ inch) cubes

100 g (3½ oz) green beans, trimmed

juice of 1 lime

red chilli slivers, to garnish

steamed jasmine rice, to serve

1 Put the coconut milk and coriander in a food processor or blender and blend until well mixed. Strain the mixture into a jug using a fine sieve and discard the coriander.

2 Heat the oil in a large wok or heavy-based saucepan until hot, add the curry paste (see below) and green chillies and stir-fry over a high heat for 2–3 minutes. Add the chicken and stir-fry for a further 5–6 minutes or until lightly browned.

3 Stir in the coconut milk mixture, stock, lime leaves, fish sauce, sugar and aubergine, then reduce the heat and simmer, uncovered, for 10–15 minutes, stirring occasionally, until the chicken is cooked through. Add the green beans and simmer for a further 2–3 minutes or until tender.

4 Remove from the heat and stir in the lime juice. Ladle into warm bowls, sprinkle with red chilli slivers and serve with jasmine rice.

Thai Green Curry Paste

Blend the following ingredients to a smooth paste in a food processor or blender: 4–6 long green chillies, chopped, 2 tablespoons chopped garlic, 2 tablespoons chopped lemon grass stalks, 4 shallots, finely chopped, 1 tablespoon finely chopped galangal or fresh root ginger, 2 teaspoons finely chopped lime leaves, 2 teaspoons ground coriander, 2 teaspoons ground cumin, 1 teaspoon white peppercorns and 1 tablespoon vegetable oil. Store in an airtight container in the refrigerator for up to 1 month.

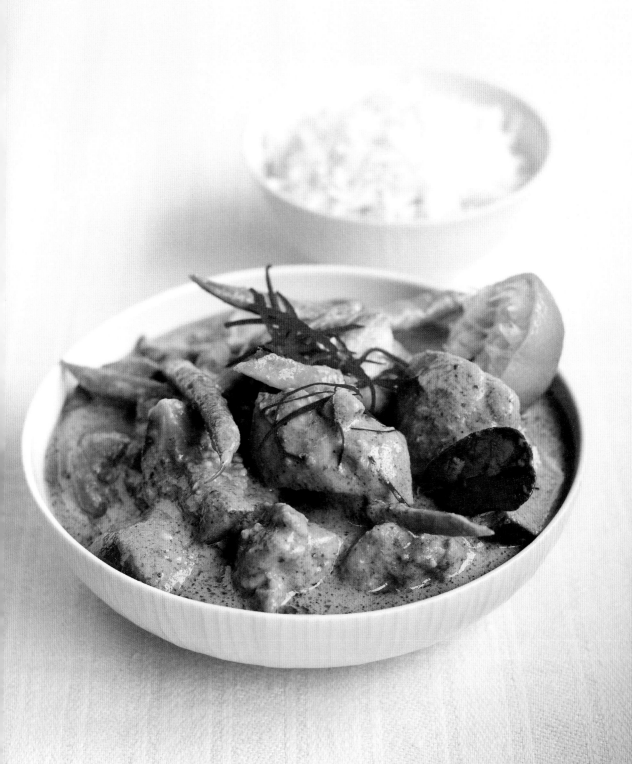

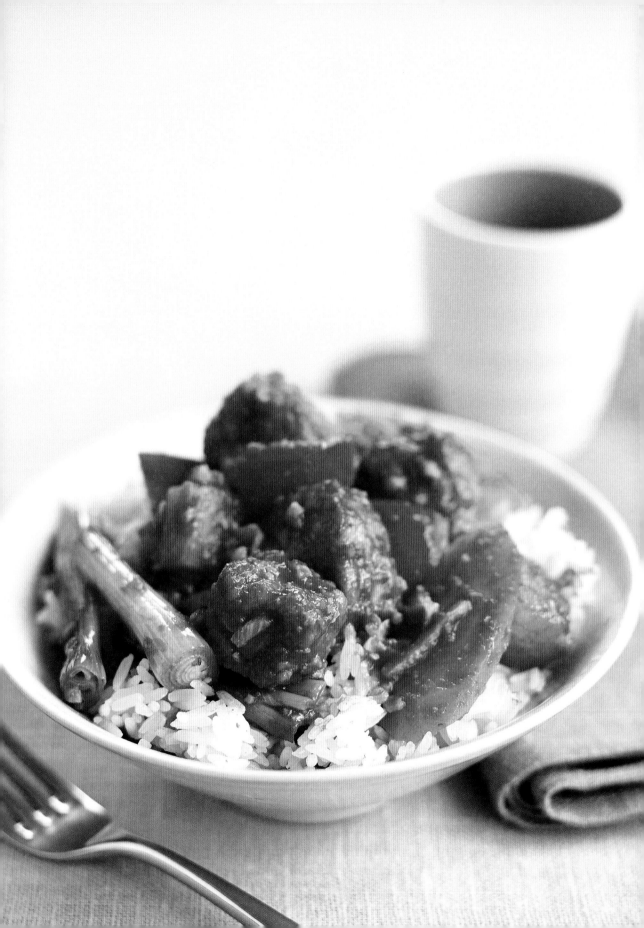

Sweet and Sour Pork

Serves 4

4 tablespoons cornflour
1 tablespoon Chinese rice wine
3 tablespoons organic soy sauce
2 teaspoons sesame oil
1 egg yolk
½ teaspoon salt
500 g (1 lb) lean pork, trimmed,
　cut in 2.5 cm (1 inch) pieces
1 red and 1 green pepper, cored,
　deseeded and cubed
1 carrot, sliced into rounds
150 g (5 oz) drained tinned
　pineapple, chopped

4 spring onions, sliced
4 tablespoons plain flour
vegetable oil, for deep-frying
cooked rice, to serve (optional)

Sweet and sour sauce
200 ml (7 fl oz) malt vinegar
100 ml (3½ fl oz) Chinese rice wine
2 tablespoons caster sugar
4 tablespoons tomato purée
1.5 cm (1 inch) piece of fresh root
　ginger, sliced
3 garlic cloves, crushed

1　Place 1 tablespoon of the cornflour in a large bowl and stir in the rice wine to make a paste, then stir in 1 tablespoon of the soy sauce, the sesame oil, egg yolk and salt. Add the pork and mix well, then cover and leave to marinate for 2 hours or up to overnight in the refrigerator.

2　Stir the ingredients for the sweet and sour sauce in a pan and bring to the boil. Add the peppers and carrot and reduce the heat. Simmer gently for 5 minutes, stir in the pineapple and cook for a further 3–4 minutes until the vegetables and fruit are tender. Stir in the remaining soy sauce and spring onions and set aside.

3　Combine the flour and remaining 3 tablespoons of cornflour and stir into the marinated pork.

4　Pour enough vegetable oil into a wok to deep-fry the pork, and heat it to 190°C (375°F), or until a cube of bread dropped into the oil turns golden in 20 seconds. Deep fry the pork in batches for 3–4 minutes, until golden. Remove using a slotted spoon and drain on kitchen paper, then toss into the sweet and sour sauce. Serve with rice, if liked.

Sweet and Sour Vegetables

Omit the pork and marinade. Make the sweet and sour sauce as above and set aside. Heat 1 tablespoon vegetable oil in a wok and stir-fry 1 sliced carrot, 1 red and 1 yellow pepper, deseeded and cut into strips, 200 g (7 oz) cauliflower florets and 5 sliced spring onions, for 3 minutes. Pour in the sauce and simmer until the vegetables are tender.

Mediterranean Roast Lamb

Serves 6

1 tablespoon chopped rosemary
2 teaspoons paprika
1.5 kg (3 lb) leg of lamb
3 tablespoons extra virgin olive oil
2 tablespoons tomato purée
2 garlic cloves, crushed
2 red onions, cut into wedges
1 fennel bulb, cut into wedges

2 red peppers, cored, deseeded and cut into chunks
2 orange or yellow peppers, cored, deseeded and cut into chunks
3 courgettes, thickly sliced
50 g (2 oz) pine nuts
300 ml (½ pint) red or white wine
salt and pepper

1 Mix the rosemary and paprika with a little salt and rub all over the surface of the lamb. Put in a large roasting pan and roast in a preheated oven, 220°C (425°F), Gas Mark 7, for 15 minutes.

2 Meanwhile, mix the oil with the tomato purée and garlic. Put all the vegetables in a bowl, add the oil mixture and toss the ingredients together until coated.

3 Reduce the oven temperature to 180°C (350°F), Gas Mark 4. Tip the vegetables into the pan around the lamb and scatter with the pine nuts and a little salt. Return to the oven for a further 1 hour. (The lamb will still be pink in the centre. If you prefer it well done, cook for an extra 20 minutes, transferring the vegetables to a serving plate if they start to become too browned.)

4 Transfer the lamb to a serving plate or board, ready to carve. Cover with foil and leave to rest for 15 minutes. Using a slotted spoon, transfer the vegetables to a serving dish and keep warm.

5 Pour the wine into the roasting pan and bring to the boil on the hob, scraping up the residue from the base. Boil for a few minutes until slightly reduced, then transfer to a small jug.

6 Serve the lamb with the wine reduction, for pouring over, and Fruited Bulgur Wheat (see below), if liked.

Fruited Bulgur Wheat

Put 375 g (12 oz) bulgur wheat into a heatproof bowl with ¼ teaspoon each ground cinnamon and nutmeg. Add 400 ml (14 fl oz) boiling water or stock, cover and leave to rest in a warm place for 20 minutes. Stir in 75 g (3 oz) each chopped dates and seedless sultanas and serve.

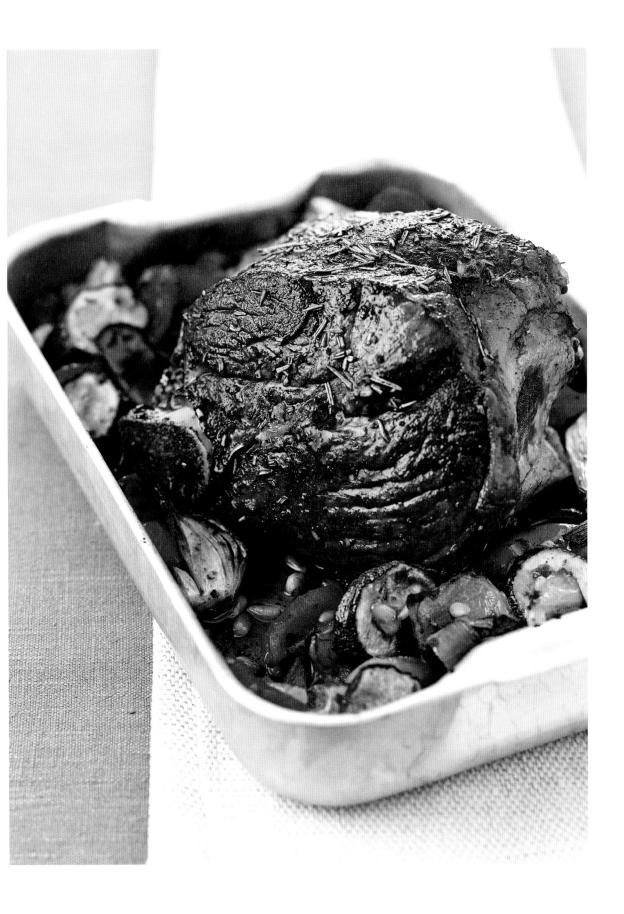

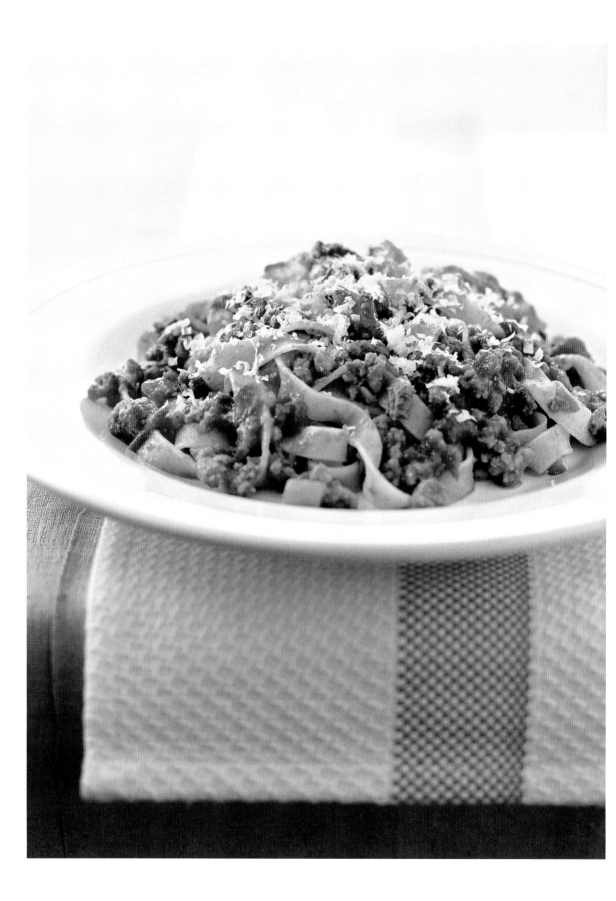

Classic Bolognese

Serves 4

25 g (1 oz) unsalted butter
1 tablespoon extra virgin olive oil
1 small onion, finely chopped
2 celery sticks, finely chopped
1 carrot, finely chopped
1 bay leaf
200 g (7 oz) lean minced beef
200 g (7 oz) lean minced pork
150 ml (¼ pint) dry white wine
150 ml (¼ pint) milk
large pinch of freshly grated nutmeg
2 × 400 g (13 oz) cans chopped
    tomatoes
400–600 ml (14 fl oz–1 pint)
    chicken stock
400 g (13 oz) fettuccine
salt and pepper
freshly grated Parmesan cheese,
    to serve

1 Melt the butter with the oil in a large, heavy-based saucepan over a low heat. Add the onion, celery, carrot and bay leaf and cook, stirring occasionally, for 10 minutes until softened but not coloured. Add the meat, season with salt and pepper and cook, stirring, over a medium heat until no longer pink.

2 Pour in the wine and bring to the boil. Gently simmer for 15 minutes until evaporated. Stir in the milk and nutmeg and simmer for a further 15 minutes until the milk has evaporated. Stir in the tomatoes and cook, uncovered, over a very low heat for 3–5 hours. The sauce will be very thick, so when it begins to stick, add 100 ml (3½ fl oz) of the stock at a time, as needed.

3 Cook the pasta in a large saucepan of salted boiling water according to the packet instructions until al dente. Drain thoroughly, reserving a ladleful of the cooking water.

4 Return to the pan and place over a low heat. Add the sauce and stir for 30 seconds, then pour in the reserved pasta cooking water and stir until the pasta is well coated and looks silky. Serve immediately with a scattering of grated Parmesan.

Beef and Lentil Chilli

Serves 4

1 tablespoon extra virgin olive oil
1 large onion, diced
2 garlic cloves, crushed
1 red pepper, cored, deseeded
   and diced
1 teaspoon chilli powder
1 teaspoon paprika
1 teaspoon ground cumin
250 g (8 oz) minced beef
400 g (13 oz) can green lentils,
   drained and rinsed
200 ml (7 fl oz) water
400 g (13 oz) can chopped tomatoes
½ teaspoon sugar
2 tablespoons tomato purée
400 g (13 oz) can kidney beans,
   drained and rinsed
cooked long grain rice, to serve

1 Heat the oil in a saucepan, add the onion and cook for 1 minute. Add the garlic and pepper and cook for 1 minute, then stir in the spices. Add the beef and cook, stirring occasionally, for 4 minutes until browned.

2 Stir in the lentils, measured water, tomatoes, sugar and tomato purée. Bring to a simmer and cook for 10–12 minutes, breaking the tomatoes up with a wooden spoon. Stir in the kidney beans and cook for 2 minutes until heated through. Serve with cooked rice.

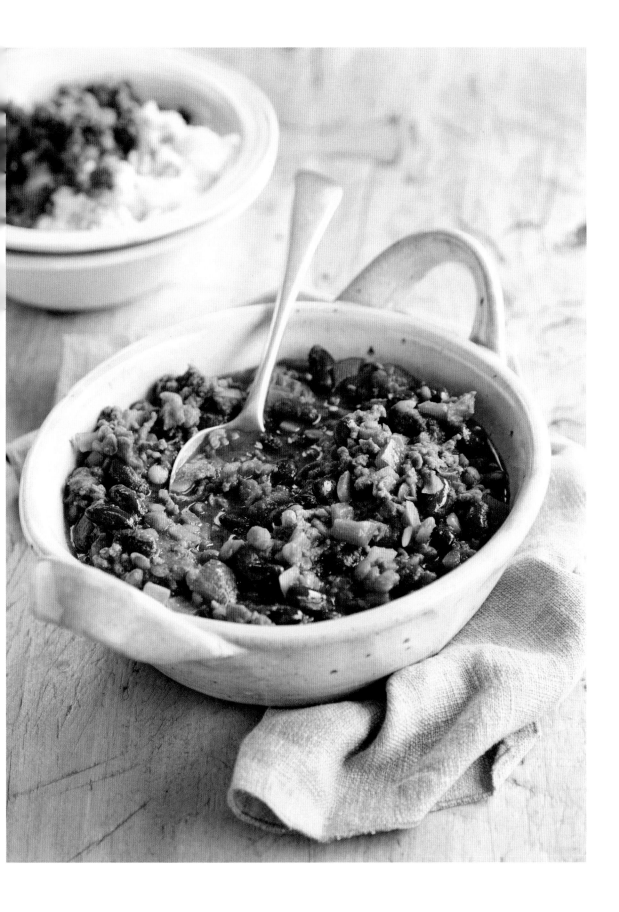

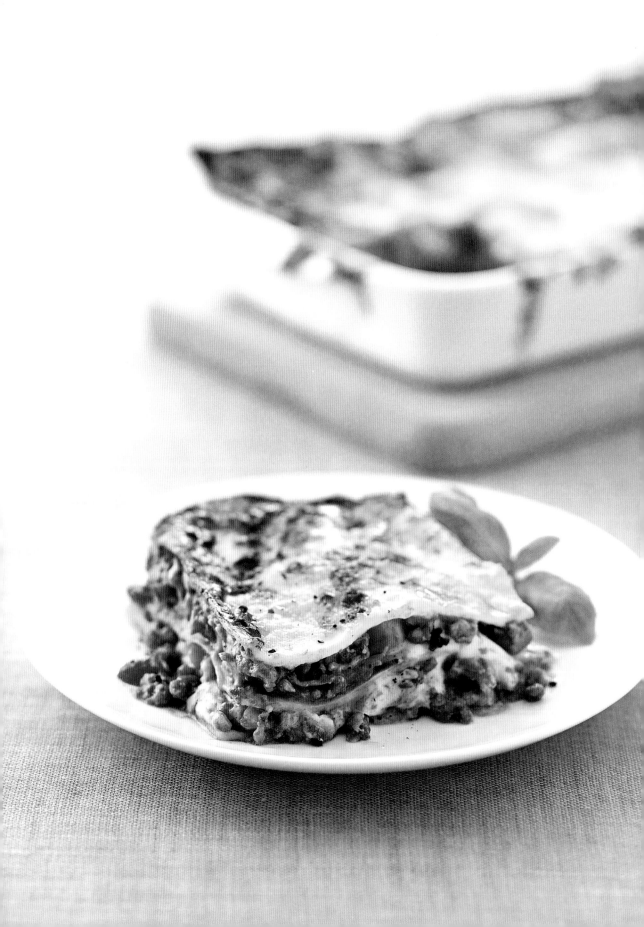

Lasagne

Serves 6–8

750 ml (1¼ pints) milk
1 bay leaf
50 g (2 oz) unsalted butter
50 g (2 oz) plain flour
large pinch of freshly grated nutmeg
1 quantity Classic Bolognese sauce
    (see page 121)
250 g (8 oz) dried lasagne sheets
5 tablespoons freshly grated
    Parmesan cheese
salt and pepper

1 Make the béchamel sauce. Bring the milk and bay leaf to a simmer then remove from the heat and set aside to infuse for 20 minutes. Strain. Melt the butter in a separate pan over a very low heat. Add the flour and cook, stirring, for 2 minutes until a light biscuity colour. Remove from the heat and slowly add the infused milk, stirring away any lumps. Return to the heat and simmer, stirring, for 2–3 minutes until creamy. Add the nutmeg and season.

2 If your bolognese sauce was made earlier, reheat in a small pan or in a microwave. Meanwhile, cook the pasta sheets, in batches, in salted boiling water according to the packet instructions until just al dente. Drain, refresh in cold water and lay on a tea towel to drain further.

3 Cover the base of an ovenproof dish with one-third of the bolognese sauce, top with a layer of pasta and cover with half of the remaining bolognese, then one-third of the béchamel sauce. Repeat with a layer of pasta, the remaining bolognese and half of the remaining béchamel sauce. Finish with the remaining pasta, then spoon over the remaining béchamel and scatter with Parmesan. Bake in a preheated oven, 220°C (425°F), Gas Mark 7, for 20 minutes until golden brown.

Desserts

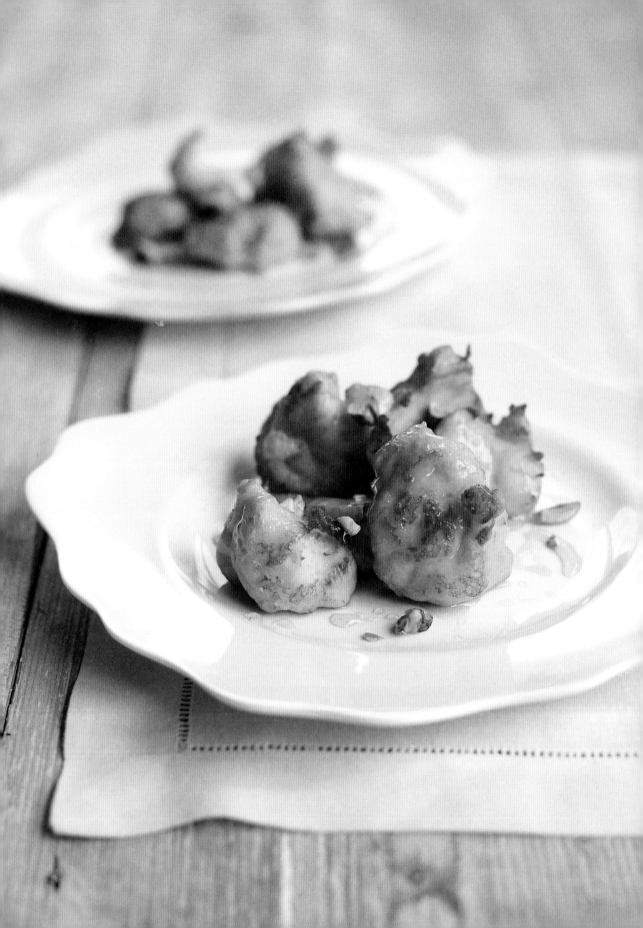

Honey Ricotta Fritters with Pistachios

Serves 4

200 g (7 oz) ricotta
1 egg, lightly beaten
50 g (2 oz) plain flour
25 g (1 oz) caster sugar
finely grated rind and juice
    of 1 unwaxed orange
vegetable oil, for frying
5 tablespoons clear honey
25 g (1 oz) pistachios, chopped
salt
Greek yogurt, to serve (optional)

1 Drain any water from the ricotta, then mix it with the egg until smooth. Stir in the flour, sugar and orange rind together with a pinch of salt.

2 Fill a large saucepan one-third full of oil and heat until a small piece of bread dropped in the oil sizzles and turns brown after 15 seconds. Drop spoonfuls of the ricotta mixture into the oil and cook for 1–2 minutes until golden and puffed. Leave to drain on kitchen paper.

3 Meanwhile, heat the orange juice and honey in a small saucepan until well combined. Place the warm fritters on serving plates and drizzle over the honey syrup. Scatter over the chopped pistachios and serve with yogurt, if liked.

Ricotta Puddings with Honey Syrup
Whisk 2 egg whites until stiff peaks form. Drain any water from 250 g (8 oz) ricotta and beat together with 2 tablespoons caster sugar and 1 teaspoon vanilla extract (optional) until smooth. Stir in a large spoonful of the egg white, then carefully fold in the remaining egg white, half at a time. Lightly grease 4 individual ramekins. Spoon the ricotta mixture into them and bake in a preheated oven, 160°C (325°F), Gas Mark 3, for 20 minutes or until a skewer inserted into the centre of a pudding comes out clean. Leave for a minute, then turn out onto serving plates. Drizzle over 4 tablespoons clear honey and scatter with some chopped pistachios.

Sticky Toffee Cakes

Serves 4

75 g (3 oz) pitted dates
125 ml (4 fl oz) water
1 teaspoon baking soda
50 g (2 oz) unsalted butter, softened,
    plus extra for greasing
75 g (3 oz) soft light brown sugar
1 egg
1 tablespoon clear honey
½ teaspoon vanilla extract (optional)
100 g (3½ oz) plain flour

Toffee sauce
50 g (2 oz) dark brown sugar
50 g (2 oz) butter
75 ml (3 fl oz) double cream

1 Grease 4 individual bundt tins or pudding moulds. Put the dates and water into a small saucepan, bring to the boil and simmer for 3 minutes. Remove from the heat and add the baking soda (which will froth up). Transfer into a container with a lid and place in the freezer to cool a little.

2 Whizz together the remaining ingredients in a food processor or blender. Add the cooled dates with the cooking liquid and process until smooth.

3 Spoon the mixture into the tins or moulds and cook in a preheated oven, 190°C (375°F), Gas Mark 5, for 20–25 minutes until the toffee cakes are just cooked through.

4 Meanwhile, make the sauce by placing all the ingredients in a small saucepan over a low heat. Stir together until smooth and the butter has melted, then keep warm. Turn the puddings out from their tins or moulds, spoon over a little sauce and serve the rest in a jug.

Tip: To avoid straying into UPF territory, it's better to use vanilla extract rather than either vanilla bean paste or vanilla flavour/essence.

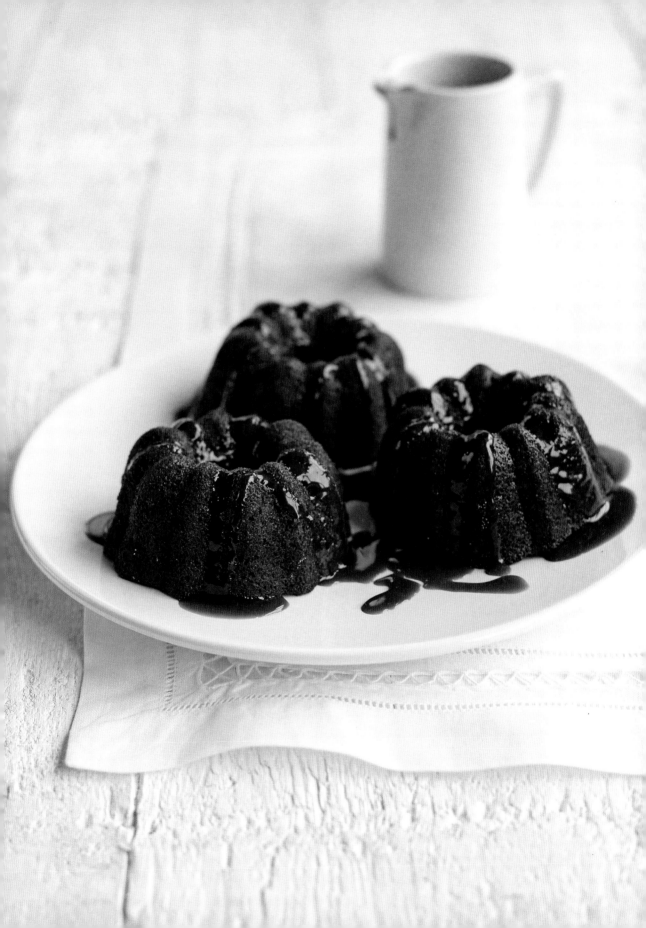

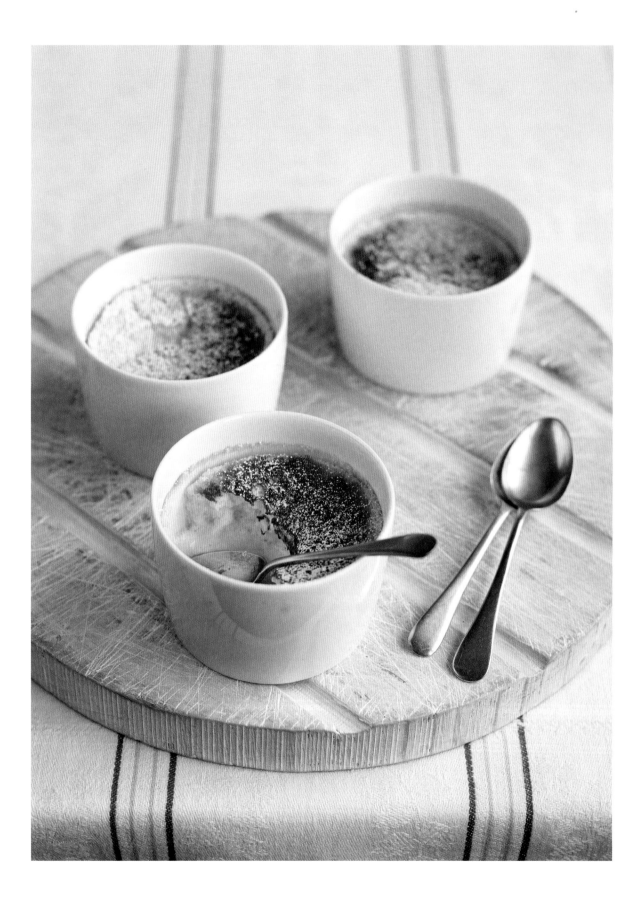

Lemon Puddings

Serves 4

50 g (2 oz) butter
125 g (4 oz) caster sugar
2 eggs, separated
50 g (2 oz) plain flour
150 ml (¼ pint) milk
150 ml (¼ pint) single cream
finely grated rind of 1 unwaxed
   lemon and juice of ½ lemon
icing sugar, to serve

1 Put the butter and sugar in a bowl and beat with a hand-held electric whisk until pale and creamy. Add the egg yolks and mix in well, then stir in the flour. Gradually whisk in the milk and cream, followed by the lemon rind and juice.

2 In a separate bowl whisk the egg whites until stiff peaks form. Stir one-third of the egg whites into the batter. Then carefully fold in the remainder of the egg whites, half at a time. Spoon the mixture into 4 individual ramekins and bake in a preheated oven, 180°C (350°F), Gas Mark 4, for 15 minutes or until golden. Dust with icing sugar to serve.

Lemon Mousse
Using a hand-held electric whisk, beat together 300 ml (½ pint) double cream, 75 g (3 oz) caster sugar and the finely grated rind of 1 unwaxed lemon. Stir in 1 tablespoon lemon juice or to taste and whisk until smooth. In a separate bowl whisk 2 egg whites until stiff peaks form. Stir a spoonful of the egg whites into the whipped cream, then carefully fold in the remainder, half at a time. Spoon into serving bowls and grate over some more unwaxed lemon rind to serve.

Frozen Berry Yogurt Ice Cream

Serves 4

400 g (13 oz) frozen mixed
   summer berries
250 g (8 oz) fat-free Greek yogurt
2 tablespoons icing sugar

1 Place half the berries, the yogurt and icing sugar in a food processor or blender and blend until fairly smooth and the berries have broken up.

2 Add the rest of the berries and pulse until they are slightly broken up but some texture remains. Place scoops of the yogurt ice cream into bowls and serve immediately.

Frozen Berry Yogurt Ice Cream Sundaes
Place 150 g (5 oz) raspberries and 1 tablespoon icing sugar in a food processor or blender and blend to make a smooth coulis, then sieve to remove the pips. Make the yogurt ice cream as above. Break up 4 meringue nests and divide half between 4 glasses. Add 1 scoop of the yogurt ice cream to each glass, then pour over a little of the coulis. Repeat the layers, finishing with the coulis. Serve immediately.

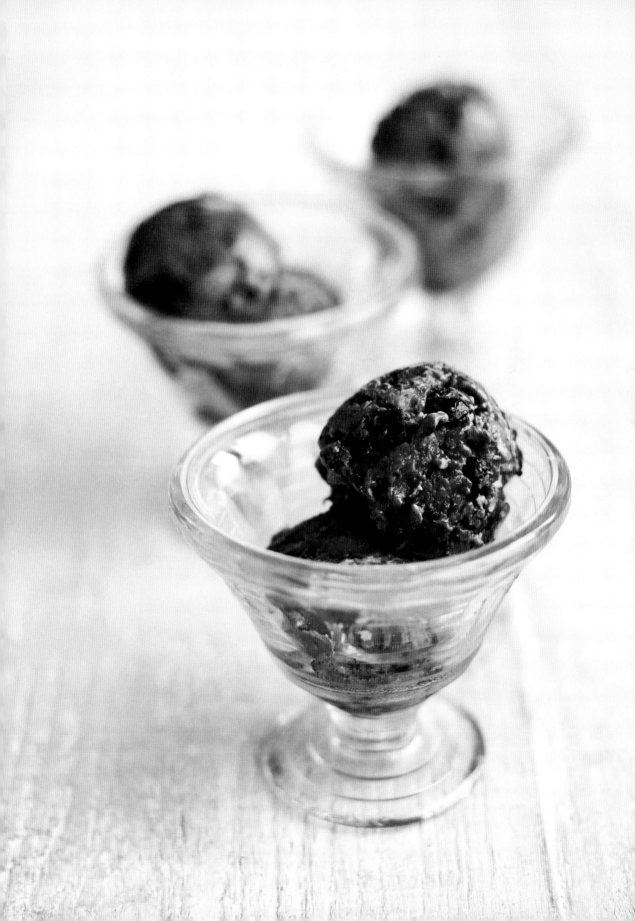

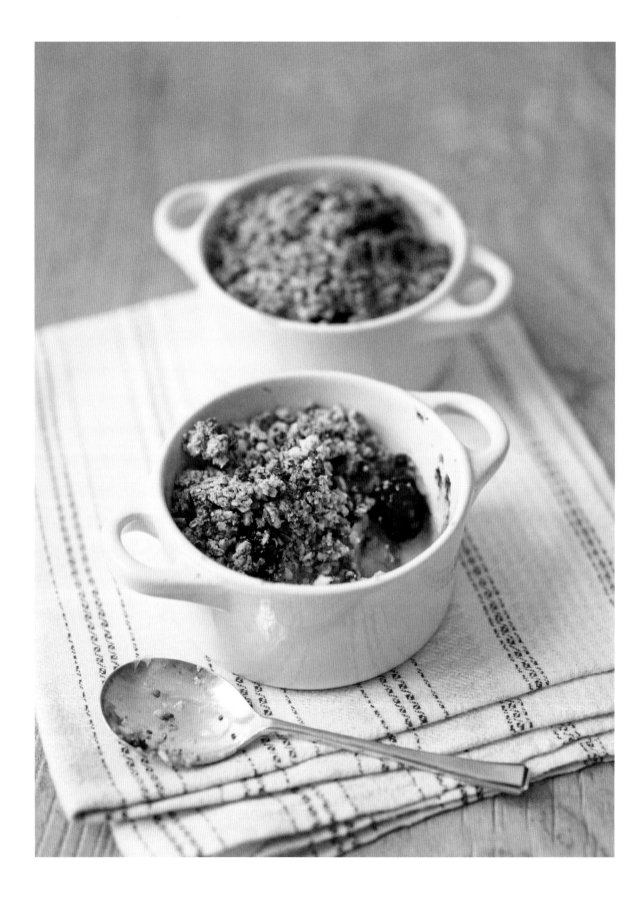

Blackberry and Apple Crumbles

Serves 4

4 dessert apples, peeled, cored
   and thinly sliced
125 g (4 oz) blackberries
2 teaspoons caster sugar
100 g (3½ oz) rolled oats
50 g (2 oz) unsalted butter, diced
40 g (1¾ oz) dark muscovado sugar
25 g (1 oz) flaked almonds

1 Divide the apple slices and blackberries between 4 small ovenproof dishes or ramekins and sprinkle with the caster sugar.

2 Blitz the oats, butter, muscovado sugar and almonds in a food processor or blender. Spoon the oat mixture over the fruit and bake in a preheated oven, 190°C (375°F), Gas Mark 5, for 22–25 minutes until golden.

Blackberry and Apple Muffins

Sift together 225 g (7½ oz) plain flour, 1 tablespoon baking powder and ½ teaspoon bicarbonate of soda. Stir in 75 g (3 oz) caster sugar and make a well in the centre. Whisk together 55 g (2 oz) melted unsalted butter, 2 eggs and 150 ml (¼ pint) milk. Add the wet ingredients to the dry and mix together gently, adding 100 g (3½ oz) blackberries and 1 peeled, cored and diced dessert apple when nearly combined – do not over mix. Divide between 12 paper muffin cases in a muffin tin and bake in a preheated oven, 200°C (400°F) Gas Mark 6, for 15 minutes until risen and golden. Cool on a wire rack or eat warm.

Sticky Orange and Cinnamon Puddings

Serves 4

100 g (3½ oz) unsalted butter,
    softened, plus extra for greasing
4 tablespoons clear honey, plus extra
    for serving
2 large oranges
100 g (3½ oz) soft brown sugar
150 g (5 oz) self-raising flour
½ teaspoon ground cinnamon
2 eggs

1 Grease 4 individual pudding moulds or ramekins and divide the honey between them.

2 Finely grate the rind of both oranges and place the rind in a food processor or blender, then use a sharp knife to remove the pith. Thickly slice 1 orange. Carefully arrange 1 orange slice at the bottom of each mould. Chop the remaining orange flesh, removing any pith or seeds, and place in the food processor or blender together with the remaining ingredients. Whizz to make a smooth batter.

3 Spoon the batter into the moulds. Place in a roasting tin half-filled with boiling water. Cover with foil and bake in a preheated oven, 180°C (350°F), Gas Mark 4, for 20–25 minutes until just cooked through. Leave in the moulds for 1 minute, then turn out onto serving plates and serve with a little more honey drizzled over, if liked.

Caramel Oranges with Cinnamon Yogurt

Heat 75 g (3 oz) soft brown sugar in a large frying pan with 75 ml (3 fl oz) double cream and 25 g (1 oz) butter until the butter has melted. Peel and thickly slice 6 oranges and add to the pan. Swirl the sauce over the oranges and cook for a further 2 minutes. Spoon out onto serving plates. Mix 150 g (5 oz) natural yogurt together with 1 teaspoon ground cinnamon and spoon over the oranges before serving.

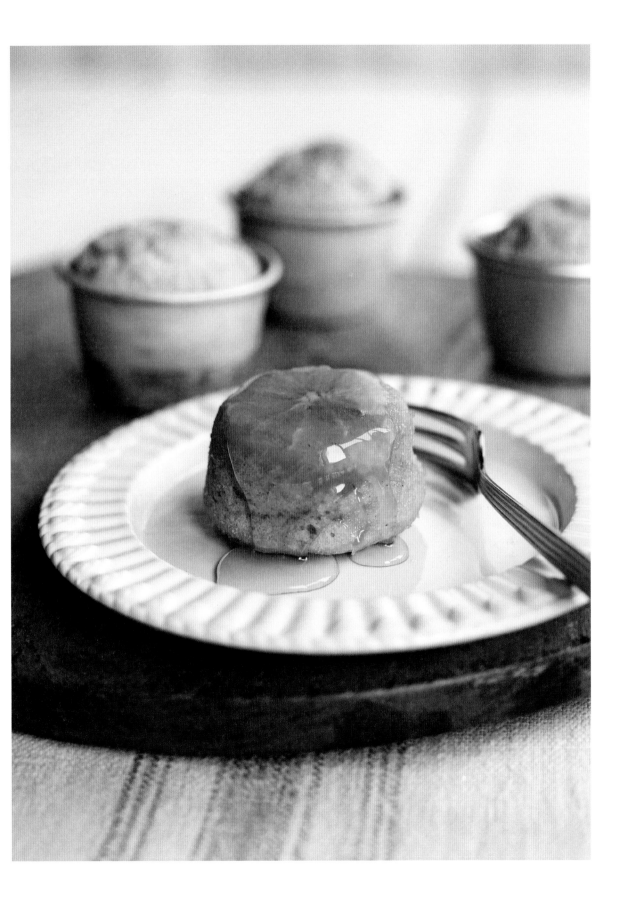

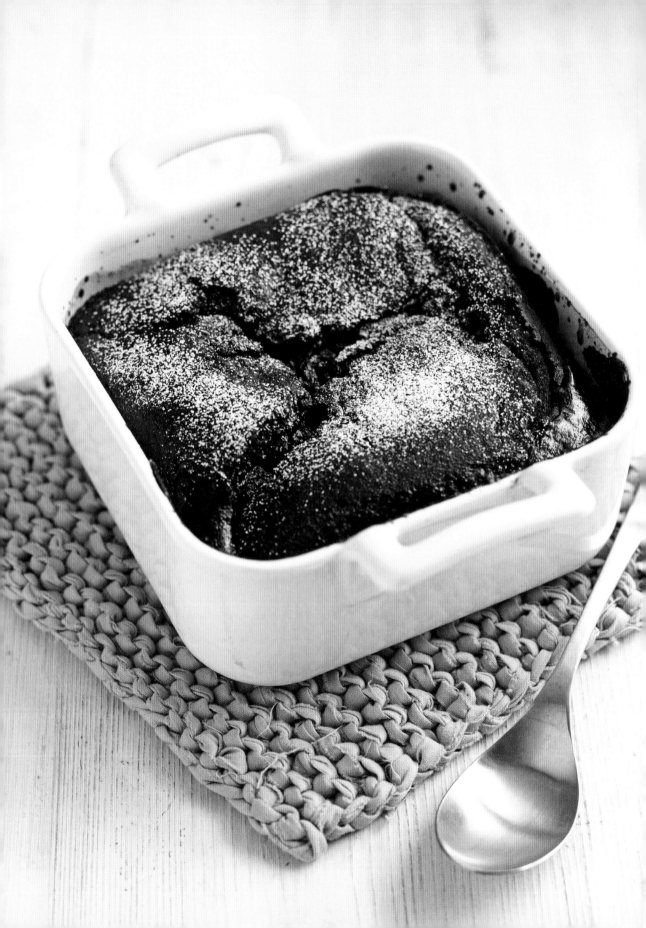

Chocolate Puddle Pudding

Serves 4

75 g (3 oz) unsalted butter, softened
75 g (3 oz) soft light brown sugar
3 eggs
65 g (2½ oz) self-raising flour
3 tablespoons cocoa or cacao powder
½ teaspoon baking powder
icing sugar, for dusting
double cream, to serve

Hot chocolate sauce
2 tablespoons cocoa or cacao powder
50 g (2 oz) soft light brown sugar
250 ml (8 fl oz) boiling water

1 Grease a 600 ml (1 pint) gratin dish with a little of the butter. Place the remaining butter, brown sugar and eggs in a large bowl and sift in the flour, cocoa or cacao powder and baking powder. Beat together until smooth. Spoon the mixture into the prepared dish and spread to level the surface.

2 For the sauce, place the cocoa or cacao powder and sugar in a bowl and mix in a little of the measured water to make a smooth paste, then add the remaining water, a little at a time, and mix until smooth.

3 Pour the sauce over the pudding mixture and place in a preheated oven, 200°C (400°F), Gas Mark 6, for 15 minutes or until the sauce has sunk to the bottom of the dish and the pudding is well risen. Dust with icing sugar and serve with cream.

Chocolate Pancakes with Hot Chocolate Sauce

In a food processor or blender, whizz together 100 g (3½ oz) plain flour, 1 tablespoon cocoa or cacao powder, 1 egg and 200 ml (7 fl oz) milk until smooth. Heat a little vegetable oil in a nonstick frying pan and cook the pancakes in batches, using 100 ml (3½ fl oz) batter at a time, over a medium–high heat for 1–2 minutes. Flip and cook on the other side. Remove and keep warm. Make the chocolate sauce as above. Serve the pancakes drizzled with the hot sauce, dusted with icing sugar and with cream on the side.

Tropical Fruit and Basil Ice Cream

Serves 4–6

450 g (14½ oz) frozen tropical
   fruits, such as mango, papaya
   and pineapple
1 tablespoon lime juice
200 g (7 oz) mascarpone cheese
2 tablespoons icing sugar
2 tablespoons chopped basil, plus
   4–6 basil sprigs, to decorate

1 Place half the fruit and the lime juice in a food processor or blender
and whizz until roughly chopped.

2 Add the mascarpone and icing sugar and blend until fairly smooth.

3 Add the remaining fruit and the basil and pulse until no large
lumps of fruit remain. Scoop into bowls and serve immediately,
decorated with basil sprigs.

Tip: Frozen fruit counts towards your five-a-day portions and a serving of this ice cream counts as one portion.

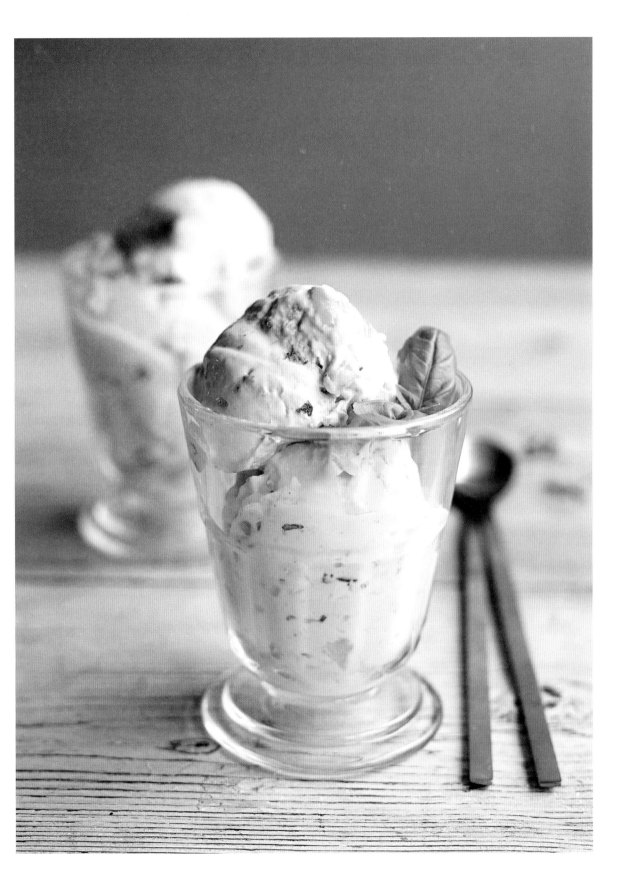

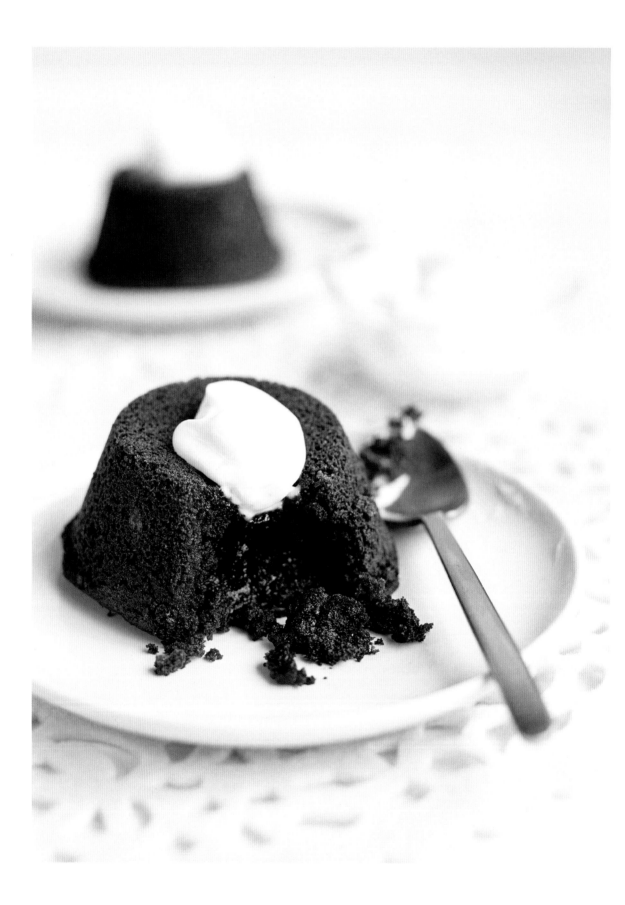

Sour Cherry Chocolate Brownie Puddings

Serves 4

75 g (3 oz) unsalted butter, softened,
   plus extra for greasing
100 g (3½ oz) soft light brown sugar
1 teaspoon vanilla extract (optional)
25 g (1 oz) cocoa or cacao powder,
   sifted
50 g (2 oz) self-raising flour, sifted
1 egg
50 g (2 oz) dried sour cherries
double cream or crème fraîche,
   to serve

1 Lightly grease 4 holes of a 6-hole nonstick muffin tin. Place the butter, sugar and vanilla extract (if using) in a bowl and beat with a hand-held electric whisk until light and fluffy.

2 Add the cocoa or cacao powder, flour and egg and whisk until combined, then stir in the sour cherries.

3 Spoon the mixture into the prepared muffin tin and place in a preheated oven, 180°C (350°F), Gas Mark 4, for 10–12 minutes or until just cooked but still soft in the centres.

4 Turn the puddings out onto serving plates and serve immediately with double cream or crème fraîche.

Cherry Clafoutis

Serves 4

butter, for greasing
32 fresh or canned cherries, pitted
4 tablespoons kirsch
3 tablespoons caster sugar
25 g (1 oz) plain flour, sifted
4 eggs, beaten
100 ml (3½ fl oz) double cream
6 tablespoons milk
½ teaspoon vanilla extract (optional)
icing sugar, for dusting (optional)

1 Grease 4 × 250 ml (8 fl oz) ramekins or ovenproof dishes and place on a baking tray. Divide the cherries evenly between the dishes and spoon 1 tablespoon of the kirsch over each.

2 Place the sugar, flour and eggs in a bowl and beat together with a hand-held electric whisk until light and well blended. Whisk in the cream, milk and vanilla extract (if using).

3 Pour the batter over the cherries and place the dishes in a preheated oven, 190°C (375°F), Gas Mark 5, for 20–25 minutes or until the batter has set. Serve immediately, dusted with icing sugar (if using).

> **Tip:** Canned cherries are usually non-UPF, but it's worth a glance at the ingredients list to check firming agents aren't included.

Mini Cherry and Almond Clafoutis
Grease 8 holes of a 12-hole nonstick muffin tin and put 4 pitted cherries in the bottom of each. Place 2 tablespoons caster sugar, 2 tablespoons plain flour and 2 eggs in a bowl and beat together with a hand-held electric whisk until blended. Whisk in 6 tablespoons double cream. Spoon the batter into the muffin tin holes and sprinkle over 2 tablespoons flaked almonds. Place in a preheated oven, 200°C (400°F), Gas Mark 6, for 12–15 minutes until risen and golden. Serve 2 clafoutis per person with a spoonful of double cream.

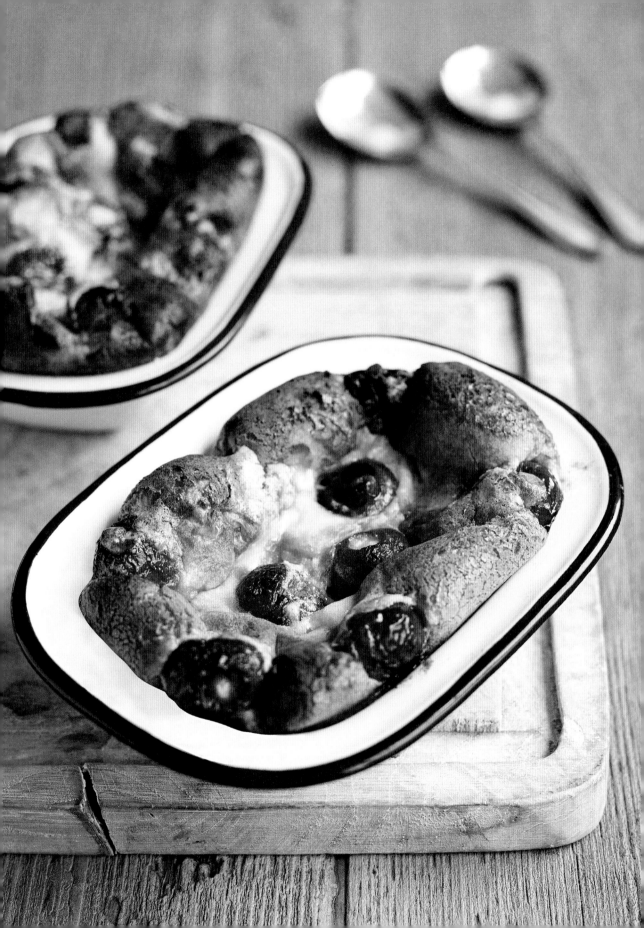

Baking

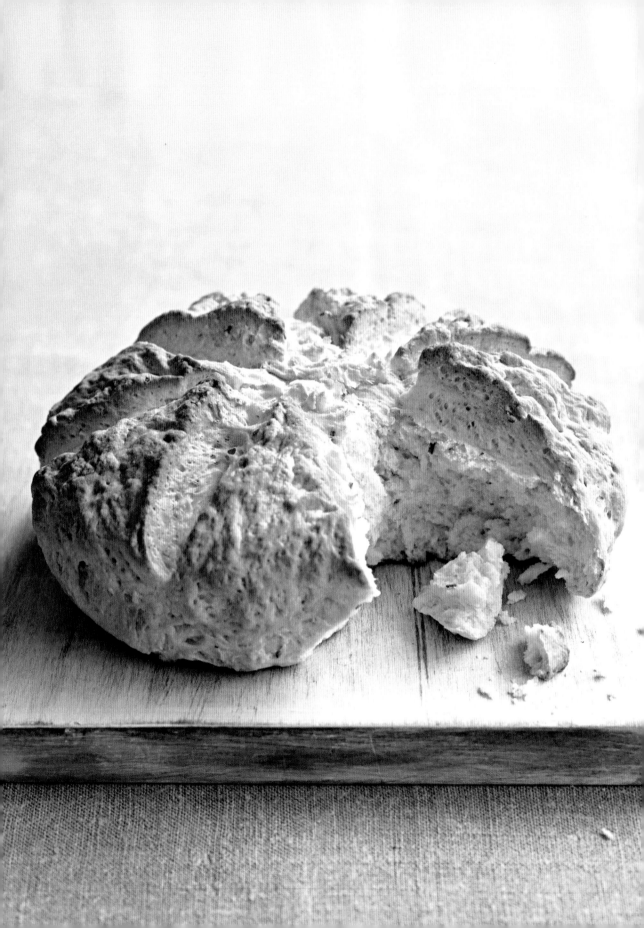

Herb and Cheese Damper

Serves 8

vegetable oil or extra virgin olive oil,
    for greasing
500 g (1 lb) self-raising flour,
    plus extra for dusting
½ teaspoon salt
15 g (½ oz) chilled salted butter, diced
50 g (2 oz) Cheddar cheese, grated
2 teaspoons chopped rosemary
150 ml (¼ pint) milk
150 ml (¼ pint) water

1 Lightly grease a baking tray with oil. Sift the flour and salt into a bowl. Add the butter and rub in with your fingertips until the mixture resembles fine breadcrumbs. Stir in the Cheddar and rosemary. Make a well in the centre, add the milk and measured water and gradually work into the flour mixture to form a soft dough.

2 Turn the dough out onto a lightly floured work surface and knead gently into a smooth ball.

3 Transfer the dough to the prepared baking tray and flatten slightly to form an 18 cm (7 inch) round. Using a sharp knife, score the surface into 8 wedges. Bake in a preheated oven, 200°C (400°F), Gas Mark 6, for about 30 minutes until risen and the loaf sounds hollow when tapped lightly on the base. Transfer to a wire rack and leave to cool completely.

Herb and Cheese Rolls

Follow the recipe above up to the end of step 1, then divide the dough into 8 pieces. Shape each piece into a ball and flatten slightly into a round. Brush each roll with a little milk and scatter over a little extra grated Cheddar. Bake at 200°C (400°F), Gas Mark 6, for 18–20 minutes until cooked.

Spiced Flatbreads

Makes 4

2 teaspoons cumin seeds

1 teaspoon coriander seeds

450 g (14½ oz) strong white bread
   flour, plus extra for dusting

7 g (¼ oz) sachet fast-action
   dried yeast (see page 18)

1 teaspoon caster sugar

1 teaspoon sea salt

1 tablespoon extra virgin olive oil

275 ml (9 fl oz) warm water

1 Toast the cumin and coriander seeds in a dry frying pan over a medium heat until aromatic, then crush with a pestle and mortar.

2 Mix together the flour, yeast, sugar, salt and toasted spices in a large bowl. Make a well in the centre, add the oil to the well and gradually stir into the flour with enough of the measured water to form a moist, pliable dough.

3 Turn the dough out onto a lightly floured surface and knead for 5 minutes until smooth and elastic. Divide into 4 balls and roll out thinly on a lightly floured surface into long oval or round shapes. Prick all over with a fork and arrange on nonstick baking trays.

4 Bake in a preheated oven, 220°C (425°F), Gas Mark 7, for 3 minutes. Turn over and bake for a further 3 minutes until golden brown. Serve immediately or wrap in a tea towel or foil to keep warm before serving.

Garlic Flatbreads

Prepare the dough as above, omitting the cumin and coriander seeds and stirring in 2 crushed garlic cloves. Shape and bake as above.

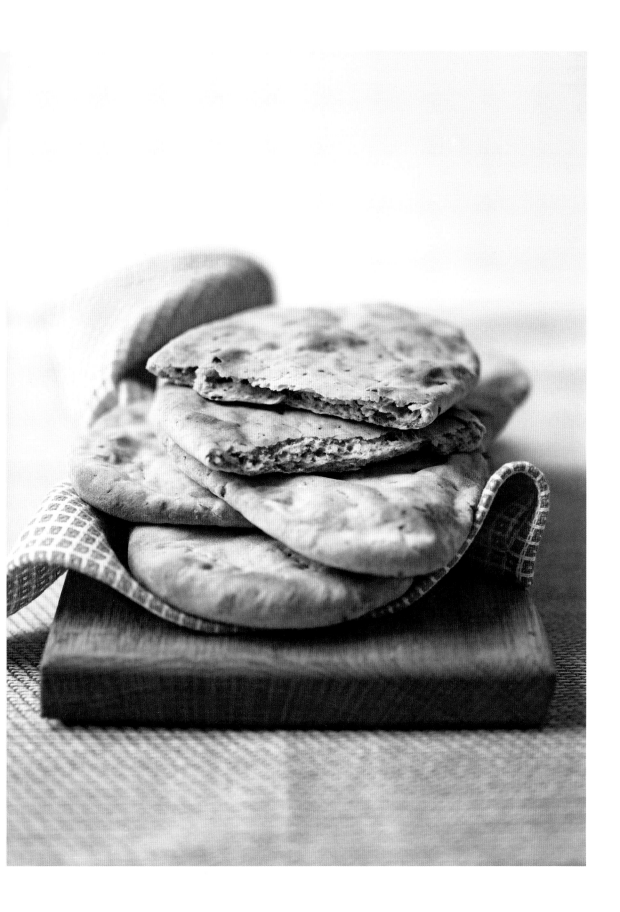

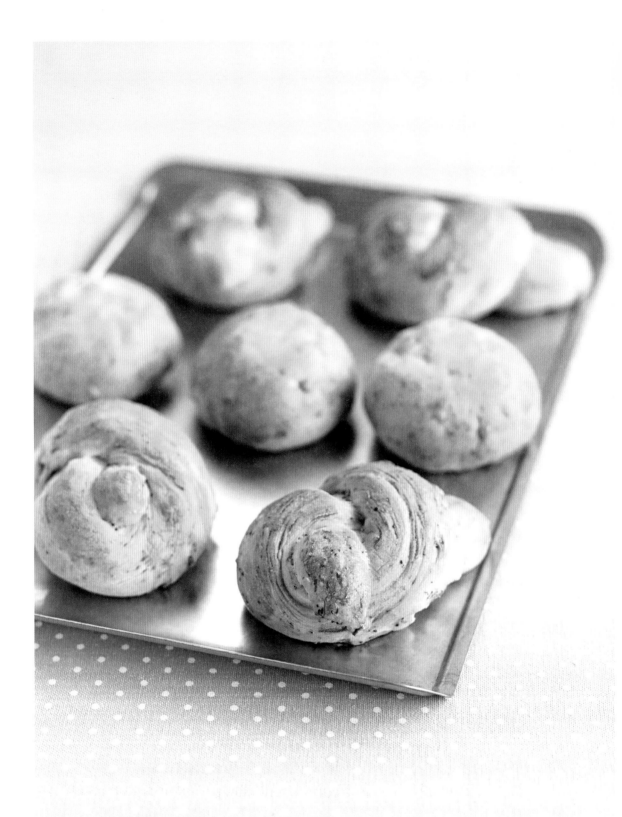

Warm Seedy Rolls

Makes 12

5 g (¼ oz) active dried yeast
(see page 18)
300 ml (½ pint) warm water (not hot)
500 g (1 lb) strong white bread flour,
plus extra for dusting
1 teaspoon salt, plus a pinch
25 g (1 oz) salted butter, cut into cubes,
plus extra for greasing

4 tablespoons sunflower seeds
2 tablespoons poppy seeds
2 tablespoons pumpkin seeds
1 egg yolk
1 tablespoon water

1 Sprinkle the yeast over the measured warm water, stir well and set aside for 10 minutes until it goes frothy. Sift the flour and salt into a large bowl and add the butter. Rub the butter into the flour until the mixture resembles fine breadcrumbs. Add the seeds and stir. Make a well in the centre and add the yeast mixture. Stir well with a wooden spoon, then use your hands to mix to a firm dough.

2 Turn the dough out onto a lightly floured surface and knead for 5 minutes until the dough feels firm, elastic and no longer sticky. Return to the bowl, cover with clingfilm and set aside in a warm place for 30 minutes until the dough has doubled in size.

3 Turn the dough out onto a lightly floured surface and knead again to knock out the air, then divide into 12 pieces. Knead each piece briefly, then form into a roll shape, or roll each piece into a long sausage shape and form into a loose knot. Place the rolls on a lightly greased baking tray, cover with a clean tea towel and set aside in a warm place for 30 minutes until almost doubled in size.

4 Mix the egg yolk in a small bowl with a pinch of salt and the measured water and brush over the rolls to glaze. Bake in a preheated oven, 200°C (400°F), Gas Mark 6, for 15–20 minutes until golden and sounding hollow when tapped lightly on the base. Remove from the oven and allow to cool a little on a wire rack. Serve warm with soup.

Cheesy Onion Rolls
Prepare the dough as above, replacing the seeds with 5 spring onions, very finely chopped and lightly cooked for just 1 minute in 1 tablespoon extra virgin olive oil. Once the rolls are glazed, sprinkle them with 3 tablespoons freshly grated Parmesan and cook as above.

Mixed Seed Soda Bread

Makes 1 small loaf

vegetable oil or extra virgin
    olive oil, for greasing
350 g (11½ oz) wholemeal plain
    flour, plus extra for dusting
    and sprinkling
50 g (2 oz) sunflower seeds
2 tablespoons poppy seeds
1 teaspoon bicarbonate of soda
1 teaspoon salt
1 teaspoon caster sugar
300 ml (½ pint) buttermilk

1 Lightly grease a baking tray with oil. Mix the flour, seeds, bicarbonate of soda, salt and sugar together in a bowl. Make a well in the centre, add the buttermilk and gradually work into the flour mixture to form a soft dough.

2 Turn the dough out onto a lightly floured work surface and knead for 5 minutes. Shape into a flattish round. Transfer to the prepared baking tray. Using a sharp knife, cut a cross in the top of the bread. Sprinkle a little extra flour over the surface.

3 Bake in a preheated oven, 230°C (450°F), Gas Mark 8, for 15 minutes, then reduce the heat to 200°C (400°F), Gas Mark 6, and bake for a further 25–30 minutes until risen and the loaf sounds hollow when tapped lightly on the base. Leave to cool completely on a wire rack.

Tip: Seeds add essential fats and minerals and also slow down the rate at which you absorb carbohydrates from bread, so you get a smoother rise in blood glucose and steadier energy levels.

Pinhead Oatmeal Soda Bread
Follow the above recipe, replacing the sunflower seeds with an equal quantity of pinhead oatmeal. Omit the poppy seeds and continue as above.

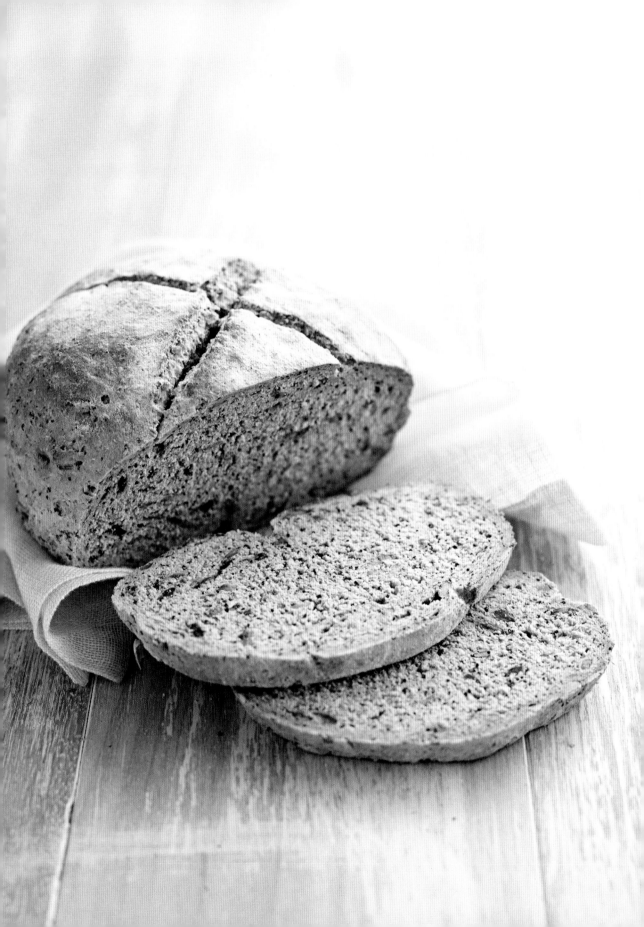

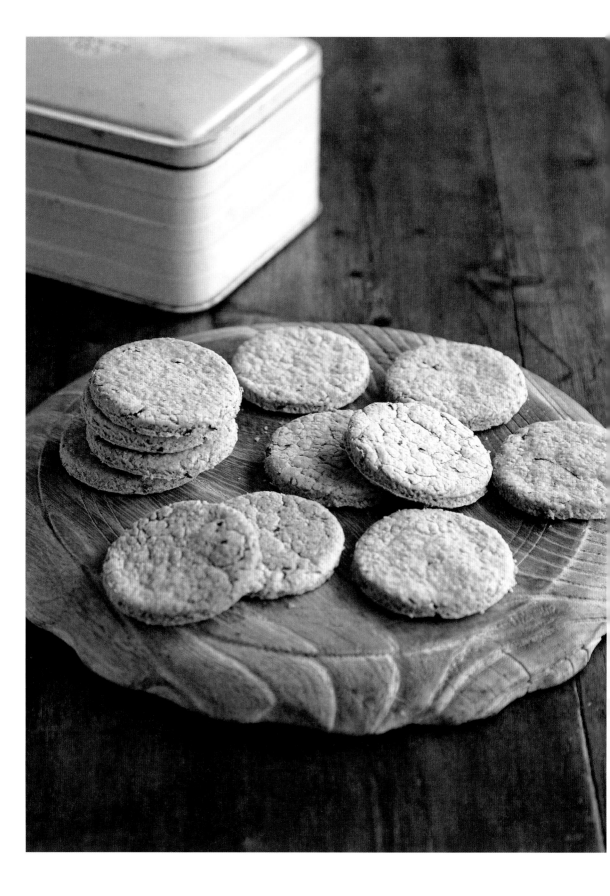

Rosemary Oatcakes

Makes 20–24

200 g (7 oz) rolled oats
3 rosemary sprigs, leaves stripped
125 g (4 oz) plain flour, plus extra
    for dusting
¾ teaspoon baking powder
75 g (3 oz) chilled unsalted
    butter, diced
100 ml (3½ fl oz) milk
salt

1 Place the oats and rosemary in a food processor or blender and process until the mixture resembles breadcrumbs. Add the flour, baking powder and a pinch of salt and blitz again. Add the butter, then process until well mixed. With the motor running, pour in the milk until the dough forms a ball.

2 Turn the dough out onto a lightly floured surface and roll out to 5 mm (¼ inch) thick. Cut out 20–24 rounds using a 5–6 cm (2–2½ inch) plain biscuit cutter, re-rolling the trimmings as necessary.

3 Place on a baking tray and bake in a preheated oven, 190°C (375°F), Gas Mark 5, for 12–15 minutes until golden at the edges. Transfer to a wire rack to cool.

Rosemary Scones
Sift together 225 g (7½ oz) self-raising flour, 1 teaspoon baking powder and a pinch of salt and pepper in a bowl. Add 40 g (1¾ oz) diced chilled salted butter and rub in with your fingertips until the mixture resembles fine breadcrumbs. Stir in 1½ tablespoons chopped rosemary and 50 g (2 oz) grated Cheddar. Add 150 ml (¼ pint) milk and mix with a palette knife to a soft dough. Turn out onto a lightly floured surface and press or roll out to 1.5 cm (¾ inch) thick. Cut out 12 rounds using a 4–5 cm (1½–2 inch) biscuit cutter, re-rolling the trimmings as necessary, and place on a baking tray. Sprinkle the tops with 50 g (2 oz) grated Cheddar. Bake in a preheated oven, 220°C (425°F), Gas Mark 7, for 8–10 minutes until golden. Transfer to a wire rack to cool.

Banana and Pecan Loaf

Serves 8–10

125 g (4 oz) unsalted butter, softened,
   plus extra for greasing
225 g (8 oz) soft light brown sugar
2 eggs
4 ripe bananas, mashed
100 ml (3½ fl oz) buttermilk
1 teaspoon vanilla extract (optional)
225 g (7½ oz) plain flour
1 teaspoon bicarbonate of soda
1 teaspoon baking powder
½ teaspoon salt
125 g (4 oz) pecan nuts, roughly
   chopped, plus 8 halves to decorate

1 Grease a 1 kg (2 lb) loaf tin. Beat the butter and sugar together in a large bowl with a hand-held electric whisk until pale and fluffy.

2 Whisk in the eggs, mashed bananas, buttermilk and vanilla extract (if using) until well combined. Sift over the flour, bicarbonate of soda, baking powder and salt and gently fold in with a large metal spoon, then stir in the chopped pecan nuts.

3 Spoon the mixture into the prepared tin and arrange the pecan halves down the centre. Bake in a preheated oven, 180°C (350°F), Gas Mark 4, for 50–60 minutes or until risen and golden brown and a skewer inserted into the centre comes out clean. Cover the top of the loaf with foil if it becomes too brown.

4 Leave the loaf to cool in the tin for a few minutes, then turn out onto a wire rack to cool completely before serving.

Banana, Sultana and Walnut Bread
Follow the recipe above, using 125 g (4 oz) chopped walnuts in place of the pecans and stirring in 125 g (4 oz) sultanas with the nuts. Arrange 8 walnut halves down the centre of the loaf and bake as above.

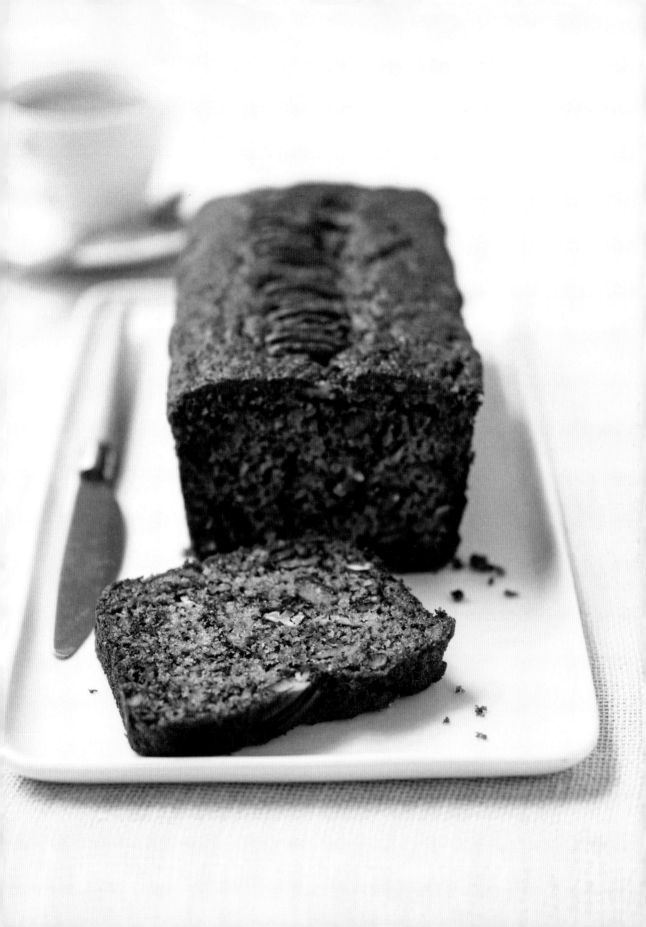

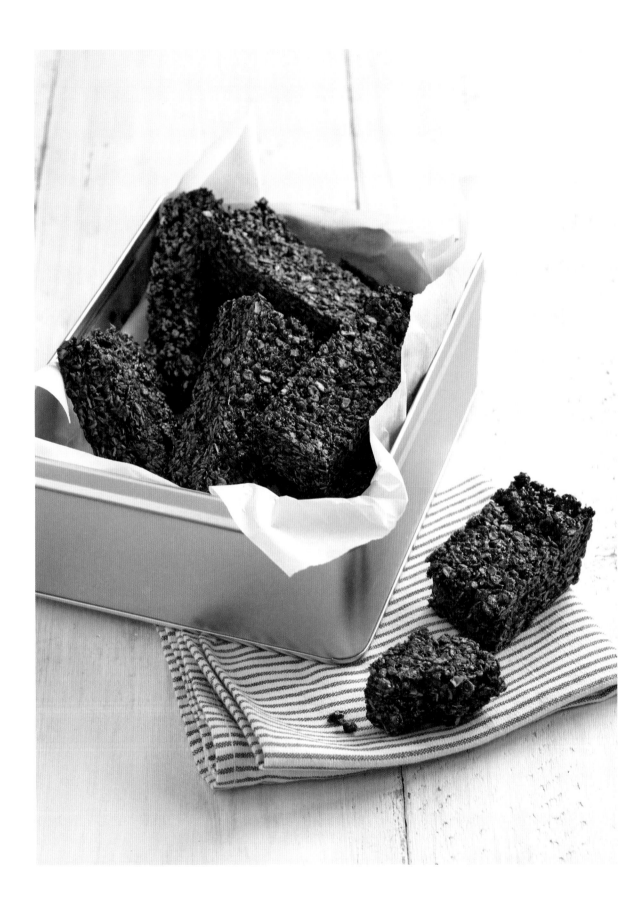

Chocolate Flapjacks

Makes 10

175 g (6 oz) unsalted butter, plus extra
   for greasing
1½ tablespoons clear honey
175 g (6 oz) light muscovado sugar
300 g (10 oz) porridge oats
3 tablespoons cocoa or cacao powder

Tip: Cocoa is a surprisingly good source of iron, which helps prevent fatigue.

1 Grease a shallow 20 cm (8 inch) square baking tin.

2 Melt the butter, honey and sugar in a saucepan over a low heat until just melted but not boiling. Remove from the heat and stir in the oats and cocoa or cacao powder.

3 Press the mixture into the prepared tin and bake in a preheated oven, 150°C (300°F), Gas Mark 2, for 20 minutes.

4 Leave to cool slightly, then cut into bars.

Peach and Brown Sugar Muffins

Makes 12

300 g (10 oz) self-raising flour
175 g (6 oz) light muscovado sugar,
    plus extra for sprinkling
½ teaspoon ground mixed spice
2 ripe peaches, stoned and
    thinly sliced
150 g (5 oz) Greek yogurt
150 ml (¼ pint) milk
1 large egg
icing sugar, for dusting

1 Line a 12-hole muffin tin with paper muffin cases.

2 Place the flour, sugar and mixed spice in a bowl. Reserve 12 peach slices, chop the remainder and add to the bowl.

3 Mix together the yogurt, milk and egg in jug and add to the dry ingredients. Lightly stir until just combined – don't overmix.

4 Spoon the mixture into the paper cases and push the reserved peach slices into the top of each muffin. Sprinkle over a little sugar and bake in a preheated oven, 190°C (375°F), Gas Mark 5, for 15–20 minutes until well risen and golden. Transfer to a wire rack to cool and dust with icing sugar before serving.

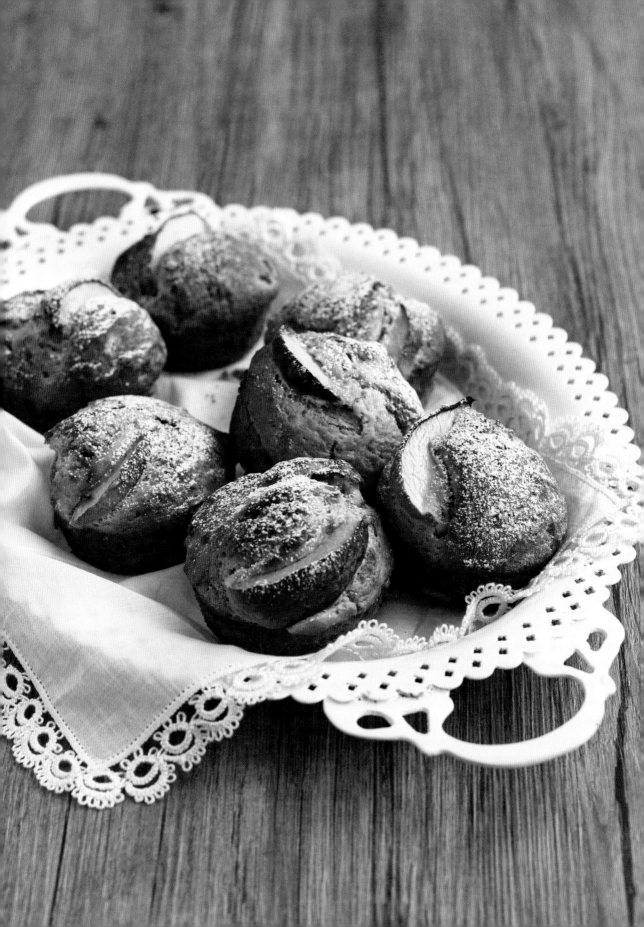

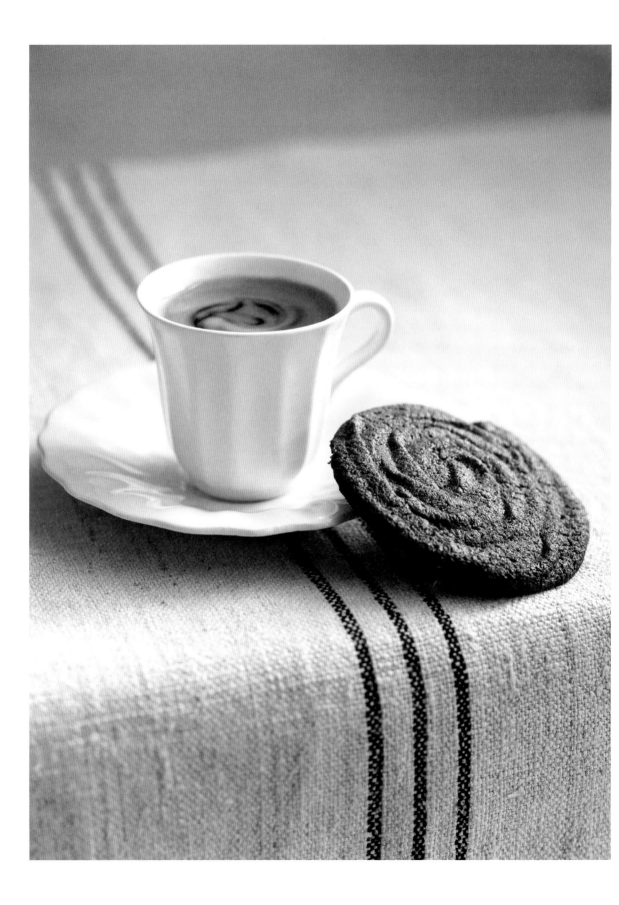

Chocolate Viennese Whirls

Makes about 15

200 g (7 oz) unsalted butter, softened
50 g (2 oz) icing sugar, sifted
125 g (4 oz) self-raising flour
2 tablespoons cocoa or cacao powder
4 tablespoons cornflour
1–3 teaspoons milk

1 Line 2 baking trays with nonstick baking paper. Place the butter and icing sugar in a bowl and beat together using a hand-held electric whisk until light and fluffy. Sift in the flour, cocoa or cacao powder and cornflour and mix to a smooth paste, adding just enough of the milk to form a piping consistency.

2 Spoon the mixture into a piping bag fitted with a star-shaped nozzle, then pipe about 15 whirls onto the prepared baking trays.

3 Bake the whirls in a preheated oven, 200°C (400°F), Gas Mark 6, for 8–10 minutes until firm. Leave to cool on the baking trays for 1 minute, then transfer to wire racks to cool completely.

Snacks and Drinks

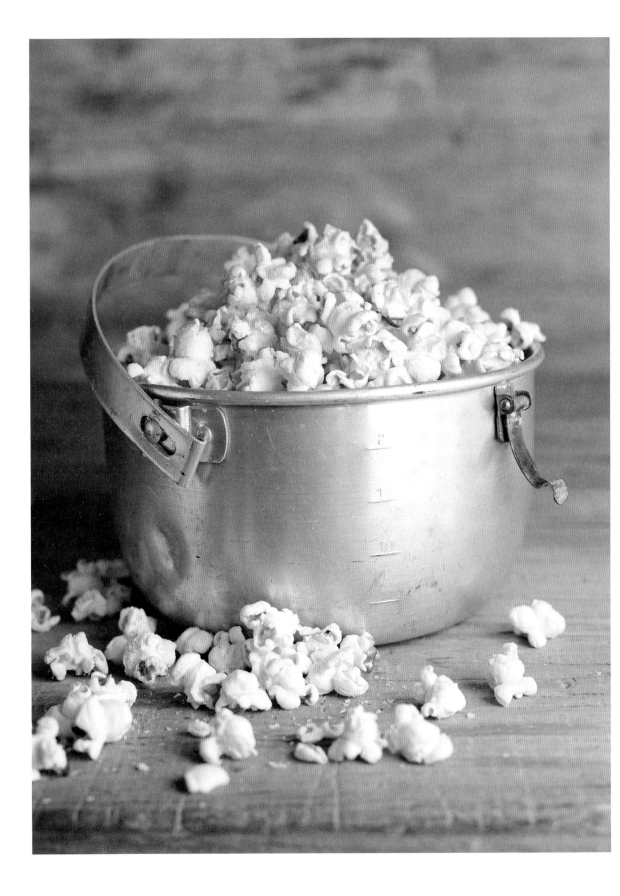

Popcorn with Chilli Oil

Serves 4

1–2 tablespoons chilli oil,
    plus extra for drizzling
200 g (7 oz) popping corn
sea salt, to taste

> **Tip:** A little good-quality chilli oil goes a long way – look for extra virgin olive oil infused with whole dried chillies, rather than added chilli extract.

1 Pour a thin layer of chilli oil into a heavy-based saucepan. Add enough corn to form a single layer in the pan – the quantity of oil and corn will vary according to the size of your pan.

2 Cover with a lid and place over a medium heat, shaking the pan occasionally as the corn pops.

3 When the popping stops, remove the lid and toss in a little salt to taste. Tip the popcorn into a bowl, finish with an extra drizzle of chilli oil and serve.

Popcorn with Chilli Honey

Place 3–4 tablespoons clear honey and 2 teaspoons finely chopped dried red chilli or 2–3 whole dried red chillies in a small saucepan and heat until the honey begins to bubble. Turn off the heat and leave to stand for 10 minutes to let the flavours mingle. Pour a thin layer of vegetable oil into a large, heavy-based saucepan. Add enough popping corn to form a single layer in the pan. Cover with a lid and place over a medium heat, shaking the pan occasionally as the corn pops. When the popping stops, remove the lid and season with salt to taste, then tip into a bowl. Reheat the honey, pour over the popcorn and serve.

Jerusalem Artichoke Crisps with Sage Salt

Serves 4

vegetable oil, for deep-frying
400 g (13 oz) Jerusalem artichokes,
  scrubbed
2 teaspoons finely chopped sage
1 tablespoon salt, preferably flaky
  sea salt

1 Heat enough oil for deep-frying in a wide, deep-sided frying pan or saucepan to 180–190°C (350–375°F), or until a cube of bread dropped into the oil turns golden in about 1 minute.

2 Slice the artichokes very thinly, using a mandoline if possible.

3 Carefully drop handfuls of the sliced artichokes into the oil, and deep-fry for about 1 minute, or until the artichokes are golden. Remove with a slotted spoon and drain on kitchen paper. Repeat with the remaining artichokes.

4 Combine the sage and salt. Tip the crisps into bowls and serve immediately, sprinkled with a pinch of the sage salt.

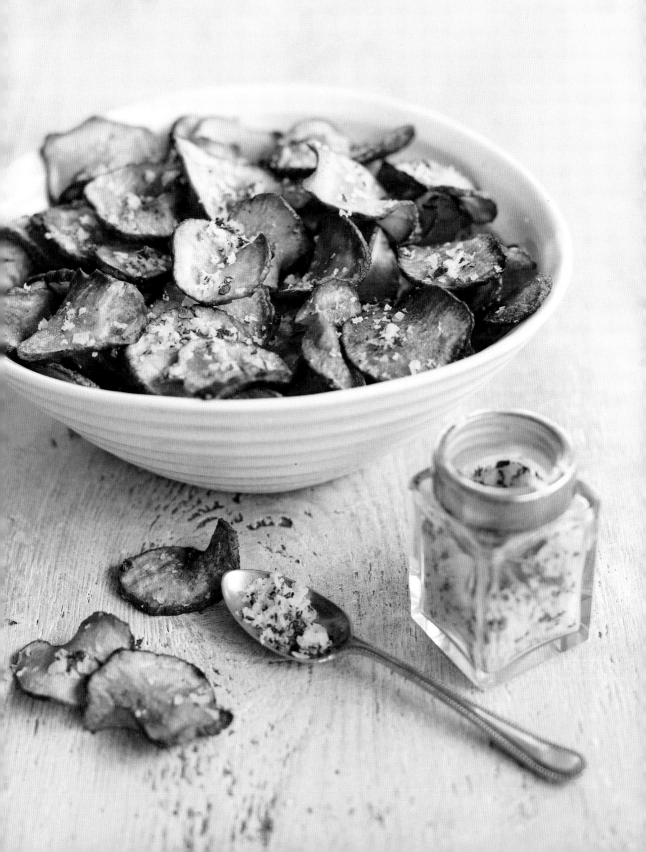

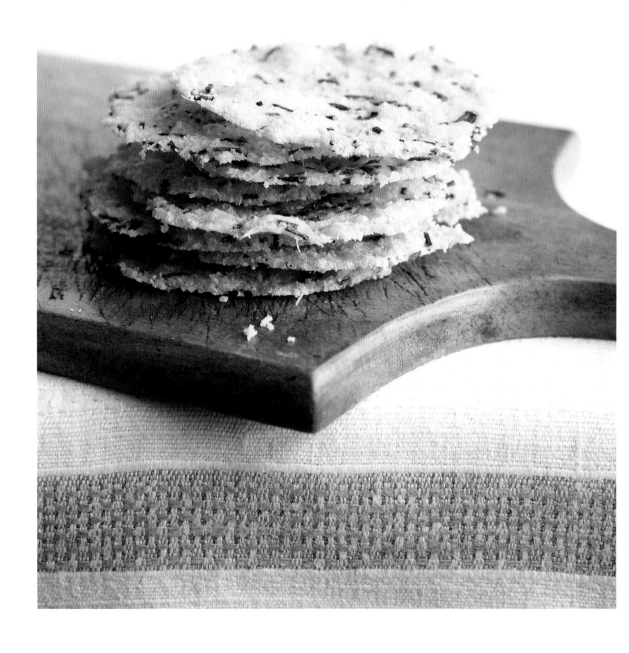

Cheese and Chive Crisps

Makes 12–15

75 g (3 oz) Parmesan cheese,
  finely grated
2 tablespoons finely chopped chives
  or 2 teaspoons dried chives
freshly ground black pepper

1 Line a large baking tray with nonstick baking paper. Mix together the Parmesan, chives and a generous pinch of black pepper in a bowl.

2 Place a 9 cm (3¾ inch) plain biscuit cutter on the prepared baking tray and evenly sprinkle 1 rounded tablespoon of the mixture inside. Remove the cutter and repeat with the remaining mixture to make 12–15 crisps.

3 Bake in a preheated oven, 200°C (400°F), Gas Mark 6, for 5–7 minutes until golden. Carefully transfer to a wire rack to cool and crisp.

Cheese and Chive Crackers
Beat together 75 g (3 oz) softened unsalted butter, 75 g (3 oz) finely grated Parmesan, 2 tablespoons finely chopped chives and a pinch of salt and pepper in a bowl. Add 125 g (4 oz) plain flour and mix to form a soft dough, adding 1–2 teaspoons milk if necessary. Wrap in clingfilm and chill for 10–15 minutes. Roll out the dough on a floured surface to 2.5 mm (⅛ inch) thick, then stamp out about 24 rounds using a 5 cm (2 inch) biscuit cutter. Place on 2 baking trays lined with nonstick baking paper, and bake in a preheated oven, 200°C (400°F), Gas Mark 6, for 10 minutes, or until lightly golden. Transfer to wire racks to cool.

Cheesy Twists

Makes about 15

50 g (2 oz) Cheddar cheese, grated
75 g (3 oz) self-raising flour, plus extra
   for dusting
½ teaspoon mustard powder
50 g (2 oz) chilled salted butter, diced
1 egg yolk

1 Line a baking tray with nonstick baking paper. Put the Cheddar into a mixing bowl, then sift the flour and mustard powder into the bowl. Add the butter and rub with your fingertips until the mixture resembles fine breadcrumbs. Add the egg yolk and stir with a wooden spoon to form a stiff dough.

2 Turn the dough out onto a well-floured surface and roll out to 5 mm (¼ inch) thick. Take a sharp knife and cut the dough into about 15 long strips, about 1 cm (½ inch) thick. Pick up each strip carefully and twist it gently before laying onto the prepared baking tray.

3 Bake the twists in a preheated oven, 220°C (425°F), Gas Mark 7, for 8–12 minutes until golden brown, then remove from the oven and allow to cool on the baking tray.

Spinach and Parmesan Twists
Place the flour in a food processor or blender with a handful of spinach leaves and whizz until fine and green in colour. Add the remaining ingredients, replacing the Cheddar with freshly grated Parmesan, then continue as above.

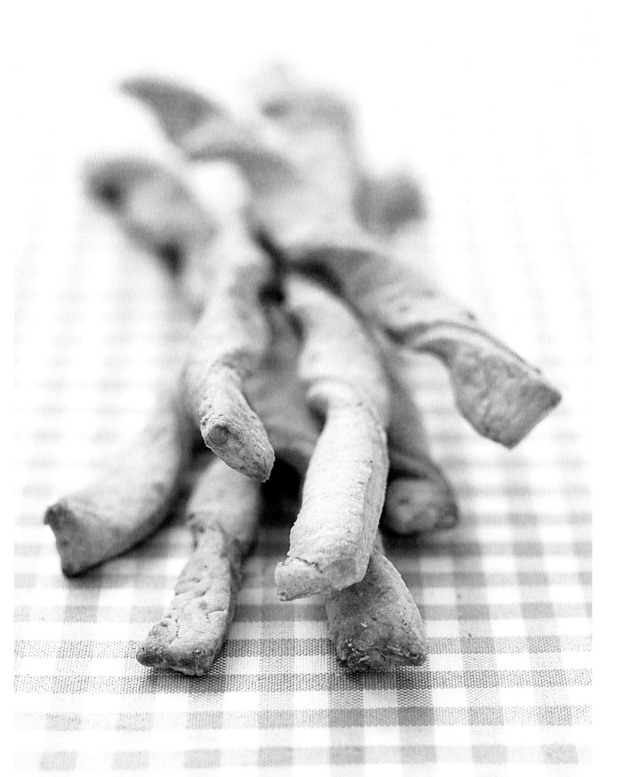

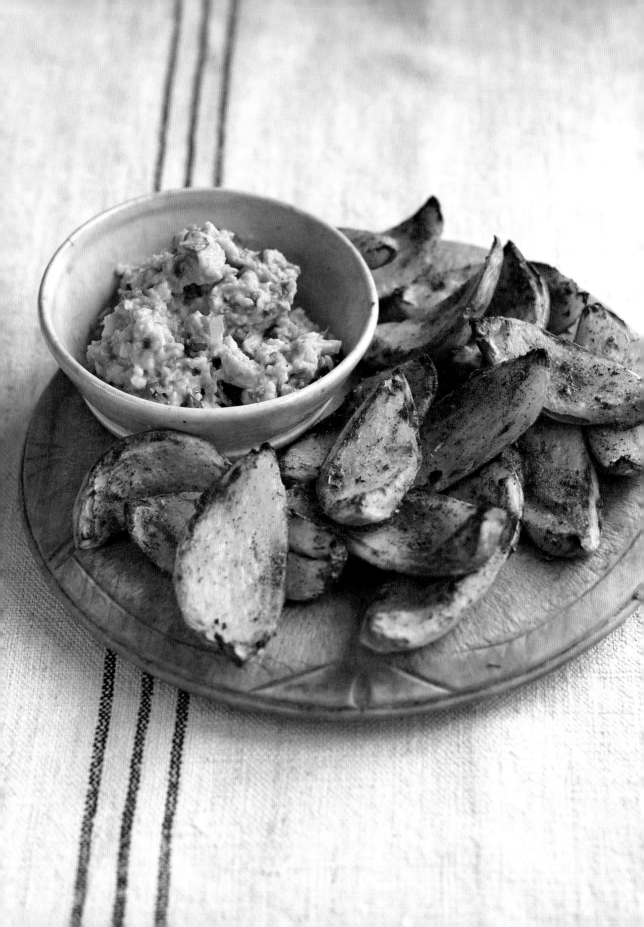

Potato Skins with Guacamole

Serves 4

6 baking potatoes, washed
4 tablespoons extra virgin olive oil
1 teaspoon chilli powder
1 avocado, halved, peeled and stoned
finely grated rind and juice of
   ½ unwaxed lemon
2 tablespoons finely chopped
   coriander
pepper

1 Prick the potatoes all over and cook for 10 minutes in a microwave on full power. Remove from the microwave, cut each in half and scoop out most of the fluffy insides, leaving a 1 cm (½ inch) border of potato next to the skin. Discard the insides (or keep it for another recipe).

2 Cut each potato skin half into 2 wedges and place on a baking tray. Mix the oil with the chilli powder and brush over the potato skins on both sides. Return to the baking tray and cook under a preheated medium grill for 5–7 minutes, then turn the skins over and cook for a further 5–7 minutes until crisp and golden.

3 Meanwhile, mash the avocado with the lemon rind and juice, season with pepper and mix in the coriander. Transfer to a small serving bowl and serve with the hot potato skins for dipping.

Fresh Lemonade

Makes 1.8 litres (3 pints)

75 g (3 oz) caster sugar
1.8 litres (3 pints) water
4 unwaxed lemons, sliced, plus
    extra slices to serve
ice cubes, to serve

1 Place the sugar in a pan with 600 ml (1 pint) of the measured water and the sliced lemons. Bring to the boil, stirring well until the sugar has dissolved.

2 Remove from the heat and add the remaining water. Stir, then set aside to cool completely.

3 Once cold, roughly crush the lemons to release the juice. Strain through a sieve, add the ice cubes, and serve in glasses decorated with slices of lemon.

Fresh Limeade
Use 6 unwaxed limes instead of the lemons, or use a mixture of the two. Try adding chopped mint as the limeade cools for an intense mint flavour. Strain as above.

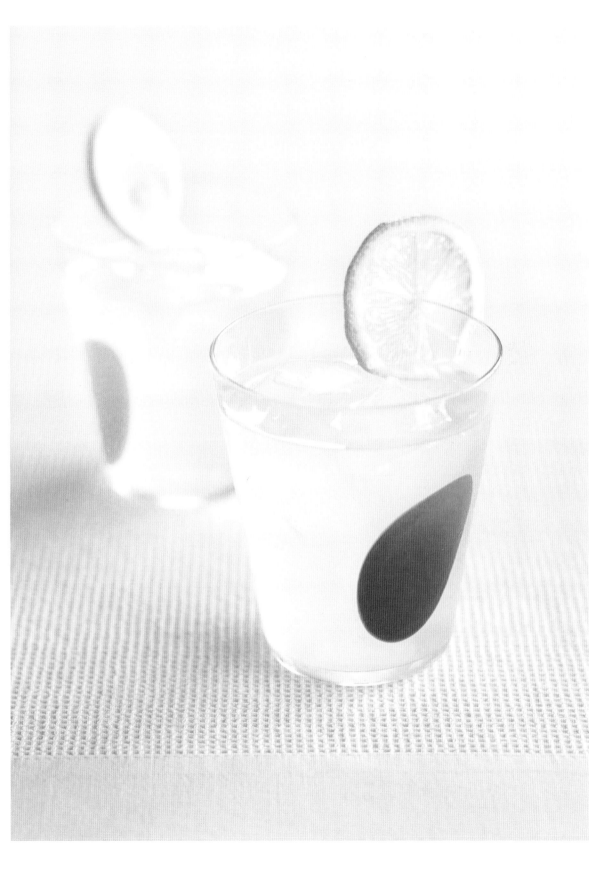

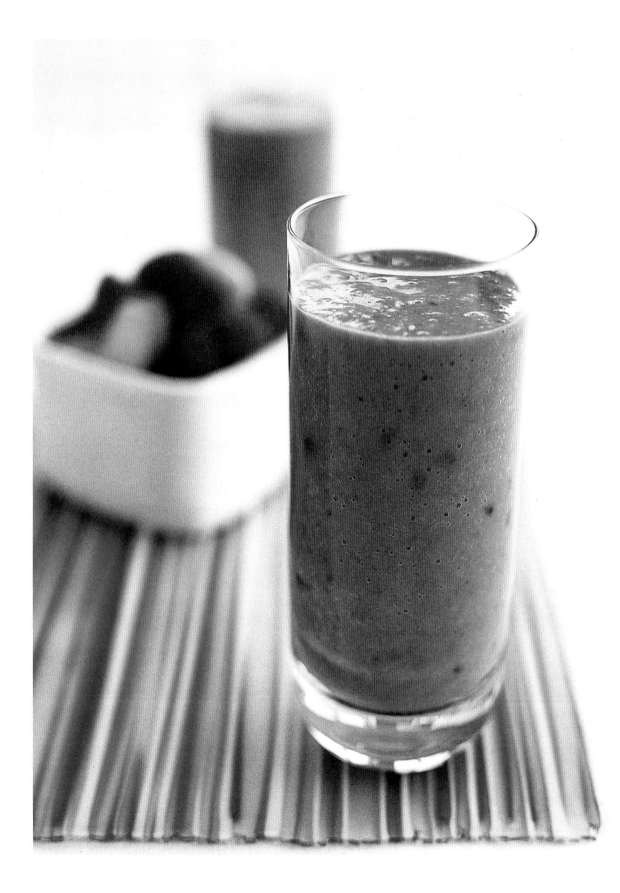

Fruity Summer Milkshake

Makes 600 ml (1 pint)

1 ripe peach, halved, stoned
   and chopped
150 g (5 oz) strawberries
150 g (5 oz) raspberries
200 ml (7 fl oz) milk
ice cubes, to serve

1 Put the peach into a food processor or blender with the strawberries and raspberries and blend to a smooth purée, scraping the mixture down from the sides of the bowl or jug if necessary.

2 Add the milk and blend again until the mixture is smooth and frothy. Add ice cubes to 2 tall glasses, pour over the milkshake and serve.

Mango Milkshake

Replace the peach, strawberries and raspberries with ½ large ripe mango and the juice of 1 orange. Purée as above, then pour in 200 ml (7 fl oz) milk, blend and serve over ice cubes.

Creamy Mango Smoothie

Serves 4

4 ripe mangoes, peeled and stoned
4 tablespoons natural yogurt
1 banana, peeled and chopped
1 litre (1¾ pints) milk
clear honey, to sweeten (optional)
ice cubes, to serve

1 Place all the ingredients except the honey and ice in a food processor or blender and blend until smooth.

2 Taste for sweetness and add honey, if required, then blend again.

3 Add ice cubes to 4 tall glasses, pour over the smoothie and serve.

Tip: With calcium, protein and antioxidants this refreshing and wholesome smoothie works well to help you refuel after exercise.

Marinated Mango Salad

In a large bowl, toss together 4 peeled, stoned and chopped mangoes, 2 peeled and segmented oranges, 150g (5 oz) blueberries and 1 tablespoon shredded mint leaves. Mix together 1 tablespoon clear honey, the rind and juice of 2 unwaxed limes and ¼ teaspoon ground cinnamon. Pour the marinade over the mango salad and leave to marinate at room temperature for 25 minutes. Serve with natural yogurt.

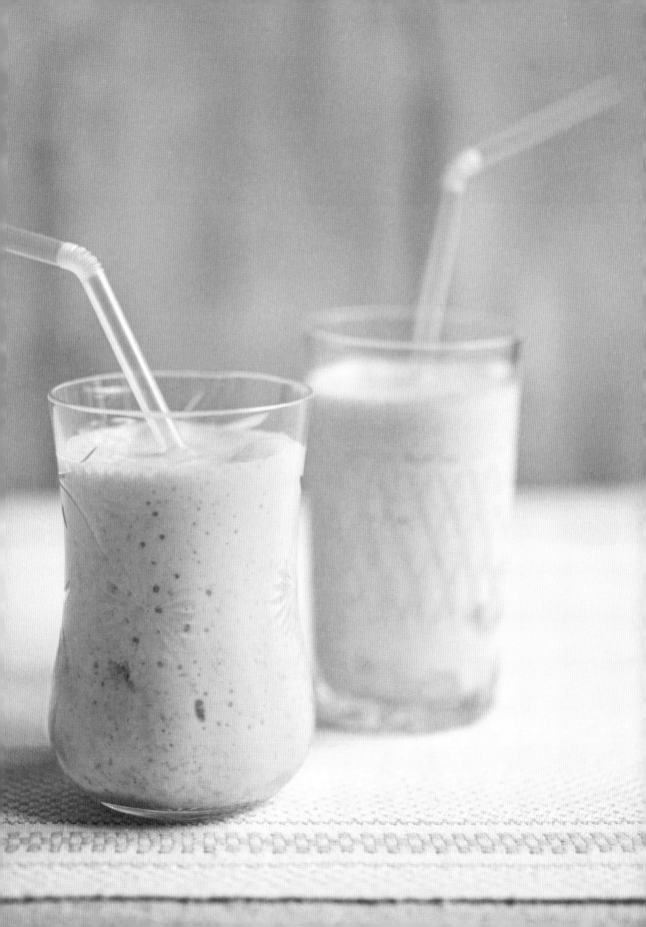

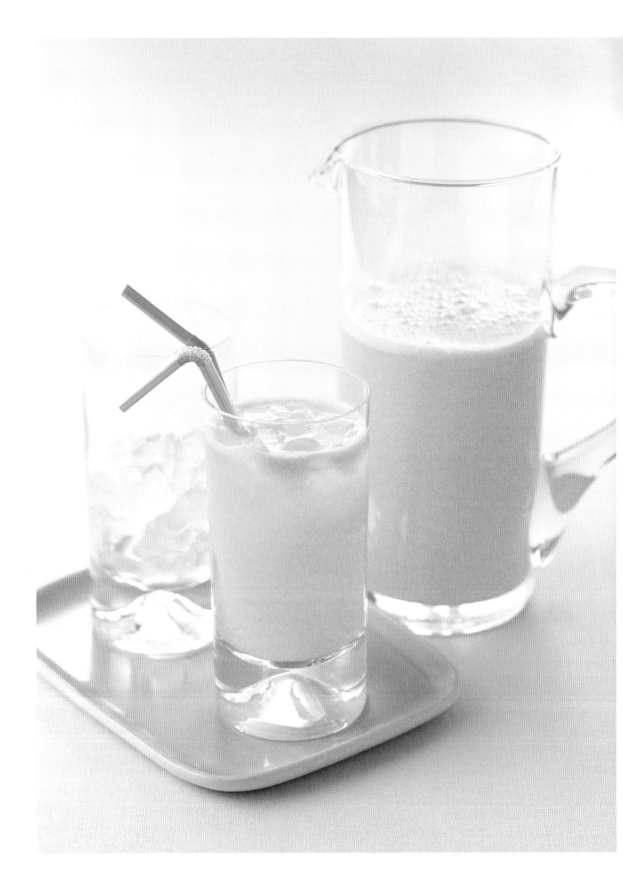

Orange and Passionfruit Sparkler

Makes 200 ml (7 fl oz)

1 passionfruit
juice of 1 large orange
100 ml (3 ½ fl oz) sparkling water
2–3 ice cubes

1 Scoop the flesh out of the passionfruit and press the pulp through a tea strainer to extract the juice.

2 Mix the passionfruit juice with the orange juice and sparkling water. Pour into glasses over ice and serve immediately.

Cherry Cranberry Fizz
Using a juicer, juice 125 g (4 oz) pitted cherries and 75 g (2 oz) cranberries. Pour the juice into a glass and top up with sparkling water.

Index

UK/US Glossary of Terms

UK	US
Aubergine	Eggplant
Baking paper	Nonstick parchment paper
Baking/roasting tin	Baking/roasting pan
Baking tray	Baking sheet
Bicarbonate of soda	Baking soda
Biscuits	Cookies
Broccoli, long-stem	Baby broccoli (broccolini)
Broad beans	Fava beans
Butter beans	Lima beans
Cake tin	Cake pan
Celery stick	Celery rib
Chickpeas	Garbanzo beans
Chilli/chillies	Chili/chiles
Chips	French fries
Clear honey	Golden honey
Coriander (fresh)	Cilantro
Cornflour	Cornstarch
Courgette	Zucchini
Cream, double/single	Cream, heavy/light
Crisps	Potato chips
Dried chilli flakes	Red pepper flakes
Egg, medium/large	Egg, large/extra-large
Flaked (nuts)	Slivered (nuts)
Foil	Aluminum foil
Flour, plain	Flour, all-purpose
Flour, self-raising	Use all-purpose flour plus 1 tsp baking powder per 125 g of flour
Frying pan	Skillet
Green beans	String beans
Griddle pan/griddle	Ridged grill pan/grill
Grill; grill rack	Broil/broiler; broiler rack
Jug	Pitcher
Kitchen paper	Paper towels
Mangetout	Snow peas
Milk/cream/yogurt, full-fat	Milk/cream/yogurt, whole
Mixed spice	Allspice
Palette knife	Metal spatula
Passata	Strained tomatoes
Pepper	Bell pepper
Piping bag	Pastry bag
Pips	Seeds
Porridge oats	Rolled oats
Prawn	Shrimp
Pulses (uncooked)	Legumes (dried beans)
Rocket	Arugula
Sieve	Strainer
Soft cheese	Cream cheese
Spring onion	Scallion
Stone (apricot/avocado/peach)	Pit (apricot/avocado/peach)
Strong bread flour	Bread flour
Sugar, caster/icing	Sugar, superfine/confectioner's
Sultanas	Golden raisins
Swede	Rutabaga
Sweetcorn	Corn
Tea towel	Dish towel
Tins	Cans
Tomato purée	Tomato paste
Wholemeal	Whole wheat
Yogurt, natural	Yogurt, plain